Made in Missouri

Disclaimers

This book is designed to provide information in regard to the subject matter covered. It is sold with the understanding that the publisher and author are not engaged in rendering legal, accounting or other professional services. If such assistance is required, the services of competent professionals in these areas should be sought.

It is not the purpose of this book to reference all the available historical records, research findings and other information in the field of inquiry discussed here. Every effort has been made to make this book as accurate as possible, based on the published information available in the areas covered only up to the printing date. However, there **may be mistakes** both typographical and in content.

The purpose of this book is to inform persons interested in the areas of community mental health policy and practices. The Causeway Publishing Company and the author shall have neither liability nor responsibility to any person or entity with respect to any loss or damage caused, or alleged to be caused, directly or indirectly by the information contained in this book.

The views presented in this book are those of the author and the persons who granted *Missouri First-Person Interviews* and are not necessarily the views of the Missouri Coalition of Community Mental Health Centers.

If you do not wish to be bound by the above, you may return this book to the publisher for a full refund.

Made in Missouri

*The Community Mental Health Movement and
Community Mental Health Centers, 1963-2003*

Paul R. Ahr, Ph.D., M.P.A.

The Altenahr Group, Ltd.
St. Louis & Miami Beach

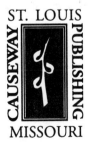

Causeway Publishing Company
St. Louis, Missouri

Made in Missouri

*The Community Mental Health Movement and
Community Mental Health Centers, 1963-2003*

by
Paul R. Ahr, Ph.D., M.P.A.

Published by: Causeway Publishing Company
PO Box 1248
Fenton, MO 63026

Library of Congress Catalogue Card Number: 2003096285

ISBN: 0-9704936-8-1

10 9 8 7 6 5 4 3 2 1

Published in the United States of America.   [MB]

To **Kathy A. Carter**, forever compassionate toward persons with a mental illness and their families, and passionate about mental health services and those who provide them.

A CKNOWLEDGEMENTS

Missourians and former Missourians, Dr. Dick Cravens, Bonnie DiFranco, Shirley Fearon, Dr. Milt Fujita, Dr. Hank Guhleman, Doug Hall, Representative Betty Hearnes and Governor Warren Hearnes, Dr. Robijn Hornstra, "Uncle" Bill Kyles, Dr. Morty Lebedun, Diane McFarland, Charles Ray, Dr. Todd Schaible, Dorn Schuffman, Dr. George Ulett, Jack Viar and Dr. Karl Wilson were selfless with their time and their timeless contributions to this book. Thanks to Andrew T. Ahr for his help in preparing their *Interviews* and this text for publication.

The staff of the Missouri Department of Mental Health graciously assisted in providing historical information and Ronda Findlay supplied key documents in the department's history, some of which she prepared at the start of her DMH career, many years ago.

Mary Johnson and the staff of the Missouri Institute of Mental Health Library rendered invaluable assistance in needed research and documentation. Paula Southman demonstrated once again her remarkable talent for editing. Dr. Robert L. Porter provided his usual gentle feedback.

Eli Lilly and Company graciously provided financial support for the preparation and publication of this book.

The quotations on pages 39, 41-42 and 45 are from *Mental Illness: Progress and Prospects* by Robert H. Felix © 1967 Columbia University Press, and are reprinted with the permission of the publisher.

TABLE OF CONTENTS

THE MISSOURI COALITION OF COMMUNITY MENTAL HEALTH CENTERS (1978-2003)

The year 2003 marks two significant anniversaries for Missourians interested in services for adults with a mental illness and children with an emotional disturbance. They are: (1) the 40th anniversary of the enactment of federal legislation establishing comprehensive community mental health centers (CMHCs); and (2) the 25th anniversary of the establishment of the Missouri Coalition of Community Mental Health Centers.

In 1963, President John F. Kennedy proposed and later signed legislation promoting a "bold new approach" to dealing with the growing numbers of persons with a mental illness for whom institutional care was the only treatment option. The first federally funded CMHCs were developed in Missouri. Today there are 22 CMHCs serving the entire state of Missouri, each a private, not-for-profit organization under the direction of community-based boards of directors. In 1978, the CMHCs in Missouri incorporated the Missouri Coalition of Community Mental Health Centers to advocate for the mental health needs of children and adults, to educate public policymakers and interested citizens on the needs of persons with a mental illness, and to promote the highest quality of clinical and administrative practices among themselves.

For the past 25 years, the Missouri Coalition of Community Mental Health Centers and its member agencies have been highly respected leaders in the ongoing fight for affordable, accessible and appropriate mental health services; active partners with the Missouri Department of Mental Health, as well as professional and citizen advocacy groups, in promoting high-quality mental health services; and competent providers of these services to persons who need them in their home communities.

Made in Missouri is tangible evidence of the Missouri Coalition of Community Mental Health Centers' ongoing commitment to public education on mental health issues. Their awareness of the importance of a book celebrating 40 years of community mental health, their cooperation in writing it, and their financial support of its preparation and production made *Made in Missouri* possible. This is a story of vision, determination, creativity, collaboration and action. This is their story.

Charles G. Ray
President and CEO
National Council for Community Behavioral Healthcare
Rockville, Maryland

FOREWORD

On October 31, 2003, persons dedicated to the appropriate and effective care and treatment of adults with a mental illness and youth with a serious emotional disturbance will commemorate the 40th anniversary of President John F. Kennedy's signing of federal legislation establishing comprehensive community mental health centers (CMHCs). This anniversary will have special meaning for all Missourians because of the pivotal role this state and its citizens played in pioneering new and effective treatments for our neighbors who experience these serious psychiatric and psychological disorders. *Made in Missouri* is a fitting testimonial to the progress made in Missouri over the past 40 years on behalf of adults with a mental illness and youth with a serious emotional disturbance.

More than a biography of CMHCs in Missouri, this book is autobiographical, built around the experiences, memories and aspirations of Missourians and former Missourians who have crafted this critical and resilient system of care. Authored and brought to press through a partnership between the Missouri Coalition of Community Mental Health Centers and The Altenahr Group, Ltd. of St. Louis, it is written from a close-up and personal perspective.

As *Made in Missouri* goes to print, the state of Missouri is facing overwhelming fiscal challenges. Beginning in the early 1980s, the CMHCs in Missouri have prevailed over tough economic conditions, while continuing to be active and effective partners with the Department of Mental Health (DMH) as we have worked to provide high-quality mental health and substance abuse services throughout the state.

In his Message to the U.S. Congress [64] introducing the CMHC program, President Kennedy wrote:

> I propose a national mental health program to assist in the inauguration of a wholly new emphasis and approach to care for the mentally ill. This approach relies primarily upon the new knowledge and new drugs acquired and developed in recent years which make it possible for most of the mentally ill to be successfully and quickly treated in their own communities and returned to a useful place in society. I am not unappreciative of the efforts undertaken by many states to improve conditions in (state) hospitals, or the dedicated work of many hospital staff members. But their task has been staggering...I am convinced that, if we apply our medical knowledge and social insights fully, all but a small portion of the mentally ill can eventually achieve a wholesome and constructive social adjustment.

Forty years later, challenges remain for mental health policy-makers, mental health professionals, other care providers and advocates. Nevertheless, the commitment of the dedicated volunteers and staff affiliated with Missouri's CMHCs has brought to fruition here in Missouri President Kennedy's dream of an America in which persons with a mental illness or serious emotional disturbance can achieve a wholesome and constructive social adjustment and maintain a useful place in society.

Dorn Schuffman, Director
Missouri Department of Mental Health
Jefferson City, Missouri

INTRODUCTION

The history of services for persons with mental illnesses and serious emotional disorders in America is conventionally marked by successive attempts to reform inadequate, inappropriate or neglectful treatment of persons suffering from these conditions. From the opening of the *Public Hospital for Persons of Insane and Disordered Minds* in Williamsburg, Virginia, 230 years ago, to the inauguration of the community mental health movement 40 years ago, each reform was a reformation of a prior reform.

To be sure, prominent elements of the prior movements, especially those that brought about public mental hospitals and mental hygiene and child guidance clinics, have continued in modified forms to the present. Likewise, the products of the community mental health movement – community mental health centers – have changed their organizational structures, community affiliations and service offerings as they have weathered budget cuts and policy changes at the national and state levels. Nevertheless, the community mental health ideology and the corresponding principles of the community mental health movement have endured, readily apparent in every CMHC in Missouri.

Over these four decades, community mental health proponents and practitioners have promulgated and pursued a progressive and practical ideology, well stated by Charles H. Frazier of the

National Mental Health Association[1] (NMHA). Testifying before the U.S. House of Representatives in favor of the Community Mental Health Centers Act of 1963, he said [38]:

> ... separation and isolation of the patient from his relatives and friends, from his place of worship, from his normal human contacts in the community actually serve to intensify his illness and to make chronic patients out of patients who might be treated and discharged in a matter of days in a community setting.

In the pages that follow, Dr. Paul R. Ahr, a longtime student of community mental health and onetime director of the Missouri Department of Mental Health (1979-1986) is joined by other Missourians and former Missourians who contributed to its history, as they detail how this ideology has guided the continuous re-formation of community mental health in practice, pursuing eight orienting principles:

1. Responsibility for a specified population
2. Focus on prevention and early intervention
3. Treating people with a mental illness in their home communities
4. Provision of a continuum of care
5. Use of multidisciplinary teams, including paraprofessionals
6. Linkages with other community organizations and agencies
7. Fiscal and program accountability
8. Citizen participation.

In 1975, Dr. Jack Zusman [111] made the following observation:

> As time goes on there are unfortunately fewer and fewer mental health professionals who have actually exper-ienced the change in treatment of the severely mentally ill from the typical life sentence in noisy, crowded, neglected wards of a state hospital stinking of human, organiza-

---

[1] At that time, this organization was known as the National Association of Mental Health. It changed its name to the National Mental Health Association (NMHA) in 1979 [54]. In this book, state and local chapters of NMHA are referred to as MHAs.

tional and structural decay to the current use of a variety of settings with graded degrees of stress and as much freedom to pursue life's interests as the individual can tolerate.

More than 20 years after the passage of the last community mental health legislation of note, there are unfortunately fewer and fewer mental health professionals who experienced the excitement of public policy and professional progress that accompanied the early days of this important movement. For those of us who have, it is our wish to transmit it, through *Made in Missouri*, to those who have not.

Members
Missouri Coalition of Community Mental Health Centers
Jefferson City, Missouri

P REFACE

Drive west from St. Louis to Kansas City on Interstate 70. About a mile after you cross the Missouri River into St. Charles, Missouri's first state capital, you will notice this historical marker:

Birthplace of the Interstate Highway System	Nation's First Interstate Started Here 1956

Just as the interstate highway system was beginning construction in the mid-1950s, the resident populations in publicly operated mental hospitals in America reached an all-time high, approaching 560,000 persons[2]. Isolated from developments in general medical, social and vocational services, in part because they were self-contained communities, the treatment at most public mental hospitals deteriorated into little more than long-term and custodial care. For many, admission to a public mental hospital was akin to entering Dante's inferno, whose portal bore the admonition:

Abandon hope all who enter here.

---

[2] According to Dr. Robert Felix [34], 1956 marked the first year in a decade in which mental hospital resident populations registered a decline.

Leo E. Kirven, Jr., M.D. [108], an observer of public mental hospitals in this era, has recorded that they were expected to be:

> ...a permanent haven for many different segments of our society, including the poor, the homeless, the unemployed, the deviant, the orphan, the aged, the antisocial, the underprivileged, the wanderer, the peculiar transient, the penniless and, at times, the mentally ill.

These conditions were to be immediately challenged and forever changed when President John F. Kennedy proposed, and then signed into law, the Mental Retardation and Community Mental Health Centers (CMHC) Act of 1963 (P.L. 88-164) and President Lyndon B. Johnson signed the Mental Health Centers Act Amendments of 1965 (P.L. 89-105).

The impact of the CMHC Act would be felt first in Missouri. Midway across the state, at Columbia, there should be a historical marker memorializing this important legislation:

Birthplace of Community Mental Health Centers	*Nation's First Federally Funded Community Mental Health Center Started Near Here 1965*

Missouri was awarded the first federal CMHC construction grant for the Mid Missouri Mental Health Center (Mid-MO). At the same time, all the way across the state in Kansas City, the Greater Kansas City Mental Health Foundation was operating a model community mental health program that had received national recognition. State legislation passed in 1964 renamed this program the Western Missouri Mental Health Center (Western Missouri or Western MO), transferring it and the Malcolm Bliss Mental Health Center (Malcolm Bliss or Bliss) in St. Louis from city to state control. Both centers were early recipients of federal CMHC grants.

Traveling eastward from Columbia back to St. Charles, you will pass through more than 150 years of the history of services for Missourians with a mental illness. Thirty miles east, you will cross

Highway 54. Go south, and you will come to Fulton, Missouri, home of the oldest public mental hospital west of the Mississippi, opened in 1851. Go north to Mexico, Missouri, where a private not-for-profit community mental health center was built in 1967, serving six counties, including the city of Fulton.

Finally, proceeding east, you come to Wentzville, Missouri, the location of the Crider Center for Mental Health. Despite its position as last in the roll call of federally funded CMHCs, the area served by this center was the site of the first U. S. foster community program, based on the program originated in Gheel, Belgium.

Like the interstate highway system, the system of community-based services for persons with a mental illness or emotional disturbance spreads far and wide throughout the small towns and big cities of this part rural, part suburban and part urban state. Just as the interstate highways radiated outward from Missouri, so too, the route to humane community-based care for persons with a mental illness or emotional disturbance in their home communities spread out from Missouri to all parts and all peoples of America.

This book is about what our national political and professional leaders envisioned for us, all of us, in the framework of what we refer to as the community mental health movement. Current and former Missourians tell the stories of its ideals and origins, the role that fellow Missourians and others have played to enhance, expand and perpetuate it against tremendous odds, and the forms it now takes, carrying out its vision for all times.

You can see this vision in action at the 22 community mental health centers across Missouri, and in the hundreds of drop-in centers, outreach clinics and transitional living sites they operate. You can hear it in the thousands of hours of therapy, consulting, education and advocacy they provide throughout this state. You can touch it everywhere; but more importantly, it will touch you if you let it.

If you haven't been touched by it yet, pull off the highway and visit a local mental health center. They are all around you in big cities like St. Louis, Kansas City and Springfield, as well as in smaller ones like Cape Girardeau, Clinton, Columbia, Festus, Hannibal, Independence, Jefferson City, Joplin, Kennett, Kirksville, Lee's Summit, Monett, North Kansas City, Park City, Poplar Bluff, Rolla, Sikeston, St. Joseph, Trenton and West Plains.

If you stop at the Crider Center for Mental Health, look for a small sign in the vestibule that will let you know that you have come to one of these special places in Missouri where the community mental health movement is alive and working. Take a minute to read it:

Abandon despair all who enter here, we offer you hope.
Abandon shame all who enter here, we offer you productivity.
Abandon distress all who enter here, we offer you help.
Abandon isolation all who enter here, we offer you community.
Embrace hope, embrace productivity, embrace help,
for you are in the embrace of your community.

Paul R. Ahr, Ph.D., M.P.A
Innsbrook, Missouri
September 20, 2003

PART I: SYSTEMS OF CARE FOR PERSONS WITH A MENTAL ILLNESS

For the past 450 years in America, the development and financing of systems of care for persons with a mental illness[3] or emotional disturbance have been predominantly a public responsibility. For the bulk of that history, state and local governments have been the primary providers of mental health services, especially services for persons with a serious mental illness.

In Chapter 1, we will review the history of public policy and action on behalf of persons with a mental illness during the period from the early 1650s to the late 1950s. The greatest share of this period – the years from 1766 to 1948 – were marked by the establishment of institutions for mental illness care by colonial, and then state, governments [4]. The proliferation of these facilities was based on the early therapeutic successes of the moral treatment movement. Unfortunately, these promising results could not be sustained with

---

[3] Over the 250 years chronicled in this book, the terms used to denote persons with a mental illness, the places where they receive services and their status in these service delivery systems have changed, each new term attempting to minimize the stigma attached to the preceding term. In this text, these persons will be referred to variously as *persons with a mental illness, patients, clients* and *consumers,* and the places where they receive inpatient psychiatric treatment will be referred to as mental hospitals, unless the context specifically suggests another term formerly in use. For an interesting discussion on the practice of changing names to minimize stigma, see Davidson [24].

21

large numbers of persons who began to fill these institutions. For a condition with few effective treatments, demands were great; resources were not.

The high rate of psychiatric and related casualties in World War II, and the battlefield innovations they spawned, generated both a sense of national urgency and a belief that the resolution of this problem may be at hand. Federal legislation in the 1940s and 1950s brought to the table the federal government as a new partner with state and local governments in the search for such a solution to this pressing social and health problem.

In Chapter 2, we will focus on the community mental health movement from the signing of the CMHC Act in 1963 until recent times. In the 1960s and 1970s, targeted federal initiatives for the prevention, treatment and rehabilitation of persons with a mental illness reached their high point in the establishment of nearly 800 community mental health centers nationwide. These centers, and their underlying public health philosophy, redefined the locus and focus of mental health interventions to the present time.

1 Systems of Care for Persons with a Mental Illness: The 1650s to the 1950s

Colonial Roots of State Systems of Care

Public responsibility for the care and treatment of persons with a mental illness in the New World dates from a 1651 letter from Roger Williams to the town council of Providence, Rhode Island, requesting that the council assume responsibility for the property and well-being of a local woman [101]:

> I crave your consideration of that lamentable object Mrs. Weston, my experience of the distempers of persons elsewhere makes me confident that (although not in all things yet) in great measure she is a distracted woman. My request is that you would be pleased to take what is left of hers into your own hand, and appoint some to order it for her supply, and it may be let publicke act of mercy to her necessities stand upon record amongst the merciful actes of a merciful town that hath received many mercies from Heaven, and remembers that we know not how soon our own wives may be widows and our children orphans, yea, and ourselves be deprived of all or most of our reason, before we goe from hence, except mercy from God of mercies prevent it.

As colonial populations expanded, such attempts at case management became unmanageable, and towns like Providence began to construct almshouses for the poor and displaced. Some persons with mental disabilities were relegated to these almshouses, others to local jails, although the living conditions at either left much to be desired in terms of humane care. Nutting [85] writes of almshouse residents that "all who were sent there went with a fixed idea, well founded, that their next removal would be to the paupers' corner of the adjacent burying ground."

Over the next 100 years, residual Old World suspicions of demonic forces at work in the lives and behaviors of persons with a mental disability gave way to more progressive understanding of their afflictions and humane approaches to their care. The influence of these modern, medically oriented techniques were reflected in Royal Governor Francis Fauquier's remarks to the Virginia House of Burgesses on November 6, 1766, when he conceived this nation's publicly financed mental illness service system:

> It is also expedient that I should also recommend to your Consideration and Humanity a poor and unhappy set of People who are deprived of their Senses and wander about the Country...Every civilized Country has a Hospital for these People, where they are confined, maintained and attended by able Physicians, to endeavor to restore them their lost Reason.

Two weeks later, the Burgesses authorized the construction of a *Public Hospital for Persons of Insane and Disordered Minds* in Williamsburg, but funding in the amount of £1,200 was delayed until 1769 [26]. The hospital admitted its first patient on October 12, 1773. During the next 150 years (1773-1923), the colonial – and soon state – governments would shoulder the responsibility of caring for persons with a mental illness in America.

THE EXPANSION OF PUBLIC MENTAL HOSPITALS

The era of sole state responsibility for persons with a mental illness started slowly. Only four public mental hospitals were built in the half-century following the opening of the Williamsburg hospital.

However, in the 60 years from 1827 until 1887 the number of hospitals increased 25-fold, to more than 125. This growth was due in great measure to the untiring efforts of a retired schoolteacher, Dorothea Dix.

Miss Dix observed the inhumane treatment given persons with a mental illness in local Massachusetts jails and poorhouses. Echoing Horace Mann's claim that "the insane are wards of the state," [26] she convinced lawmakers that local governments were incapable of caring for persons with a mental illness. In 1843, the Massachusetts legislature voted to terminate local responsibility for these persons and make them wards of the Commonwealth. Governors and legislators in other states heard Miss Dix's call for reform and assumed responsibility for the care of persons with a mental illness.

Early public mental health facilities were developed according to a philosophy of humane care known as moral treatment. Small in size and typically set in bucolic settings away from the pressures of city life, moral treatment asylums were adequately staffed and offered a therapeutic environment with active treatment that included vocational training and recreation. Success rates were high. In 1842, Charles Dickens [27] observed moral treatment principles in practice when he visited the Boston Hospital for the Insane[4]. He described conditions at the hospital as:

> ...admirably conducted on those enlightened principles of conciliation and kindness which twenty years ago would have been worse than heretical. Each ward in this institution is shaped like a long gallery or hall, with the dormitories of the patients opening from it on either hand. Here they work, read, play at skittles, and other games; and when the weather does not admit of their taking exercises out of doors, pass the day together ... Every patient in this

---

[4] It is instructive to contrast this standard of care at public mental health institutions at the time that the future Fulton State Hospital was developed in Missouri (1847-1851), with the conditions at that same facility a century later that were described to Dr. George Ulett by Fulton's superintendent [see p. 78].

asylum sits down to dinner every day with a knife and fork; and in the midst of them sits [the superintendent] ... At every meal, moral influence alone restrains the more violent among them from cutting the throats of the rest; but the effect of that influence is reduced to an absolute certainty, and is found, even as a means of restraint, to say nothing of it as a means of cure, a hundred times more efficacious than all the straitwaiscoats, fetters and handcuffs, that ignorance, prejudice, and cruelty have manufactured since the creation of the world.

Buoyed by the success of the moral treatment institutions, Dorothea Dix worked for the passage of the 12,225,000 Acre Act. This bill proposed that the federal government grant to the states 10 million acres of land for bettering the conditions of care for persons with a mental illness. First introduced in 1848, the bill was predicated on the then current practice of making land grants to the states to improve public education, as well as on Miss Dix's revised assertion that persons with a mental illness were "through the providence of God...wards of the nation, claimants on the sympathy and care of the public." [26] Although passed by Congress, President Franklin Pierce vetoed the bill in 1854, arguing that the legislation would usurp the states' responsibilities for persons with a mental illness. In the short period of 11 years (1843-1854), local governments were deemed unable and the federal government proved unwilling to assume responsibility of the proper care of persons with a mental illness. States became solely and unequivocally responsible for their treatment.

The eventual demise of the moral treatment movement can be traced to the period after the Civil War when there were both an influx of immigrants in America, creating additional demand for mental health care[5], and inadequate funding for the facilities needed to provide this care. According to Brand [11]:

---

[5] Bockoven [9] notes that, as the number of indigent immigrants increased in state mental hospitals, a new diagnostic category was developed and applied to many of them: *foreign insane pauperism.*

By the close of the century...the maxim of no more than 250 patients in any mental hospital — a rule formulated by Dr. Thomas A. Kirkbride (1809-1883) and adopted in 1851 by the Association of Medical Superintendents — had been abandoned because of the explosive population growth and great increase of psychotic patients in the United States. From the crowded slums of the great industrial cities there were dispatched to isolated state hospitals thousands unable to cope with the stresses of living. Individual treatment disappeared under conditions of impersonal herding, loss of identity and routine use of physical restraints.

During the late 19th century, the practice of psychiatry was also changing. Seeking to be identified more closely with the medical disciplines, psychiatry abandoned its moral treatment roots and sought organic causes and cures for mental illness. From this perspective, chronic mental illness was seen as a degenerative disorder, providing little prospect for recovery. This point of view was adopted by policymakers to justify the inadequate funding provided for mental hospital care. As a result of these forces, between the mid-1850s and the mid-1950s, state-operated asylums evolved from small, treatment-oriented facilities into large custodial care institutions, labeled "total institutions" by sociologists and "warehouses" by cynics [2].

EARLY 20TH CENTURY REFORMS

In the first decade of the 20th century, the impact of two persons, one American, the other Austrian, held forth promise for a reformation of the 19th century reform movement. Clifford Beers was a successful Wall Street executive who attempted suicide in 1901. After hospitalization in several private and public mental hospitals, he recovered and wrote of his experiences in a book entitled, *The Mind That Found Itself* [7]. Beers spearheaded the establishment of the National Committee for Mental Hygiene, a precursor of the NMHA.

In 1909, Sigmund Freud delivered at Clark University in Worcester, Massachusetts, a series of lectures on psychoanalysis that engendered great enthusiasm throughout America. Freud's concepts of the effects of early childhood experiences on personality development were very compatible with the National Committee's interest in promoting mental hygiene. In time, the fusion of Freud's concepts and the National Committee's agenda led to the establishment in the United States in the early 1920s of mental hygiene clinics and child guidance clinics. These clinics were financed initially by philanthropic organizations and later by state and local governments.

Eighty years after Dorothea Dix had convinced the Massachusetts legislature that local communities were incapable of caring for persons with a mental illness, state and local authorities began collaborating with local mental hygiene advocates and mental health professionals, to develop and maintain community-based mental hygiene clinics. This partnership was quite productive. According to Dr. Robert H. Felix, [34] the first director of the National Institute of Mental Health (NIMH), by 1946 there were slightly more than 800 mental health clinics in the United States. By 1950, there were more than 1,200, of which three-quarters were supported locally and without federal assistance.

THE NATIONAL MENTAL HEALTH ACT OF 1946

Despite the good intentions of the mental hygiene movement, the rates of mental illness and the conditions of care for persons with a serious mental illness were not significantly affected. By World War II, it became evident that the treatment concepts and services developed since 1773 had not been very successful. During the war years, about 1.1 million out of 4.8 million men were rejected as unfit for military service for mental or neurological disorders and 40% of military medical discharges were for psychiatric reasons. In 1946, 60% of the patients under the care of the Veterans Administration were hospitalized for psychiatric reasons [10].

The high rates of psychiatric casualties during World War II had an unanticipated impact on the development of services for persons with a mental illness. Prior to the war, such persons were often the objects of pity or fear. After the war, the presence of heroic servicemen who suffered war-related psychiatric casualties pro-voked genuine sympathy and concern for the availability of effective treatments. Brand [10] describes the effect of a Marine Captain, who had been successfully hospitalized for psychiatric problems, on Senate hearings on the National Mental Health Act:

> Offering the testimony on his own initiative, the young flyer's words carried no self-pity, but an unquestionable sincerity of interest in the need for active treatment programs for the mentally ill. His statement moved his audience deeply.

Coincidentally, the high rate of psychiatric casualties forced the military medical departments to experiment with new forms of intervention, including prompt diagnosis and intensive treatments, such as group therapy, hypnosis and sedation [89].

Two important byproducts of the high rate of psychiatric casual-ties of World War II were the promise of effective treatments and the interest of the federal government in addressing both the prob-lem and its solution. After the war, many members of Congress, disturbed by the high psychiatric rejection and casualty rates, set out to curb what they feared was a mental illness epidemic. A remedy was soon at hand. Congress passed the Public Health Service Act of 1944 (P.L. 78-410), which broadened the powers of the Public Health Service and authorized general assistance to the states for the establishment of local health programs. Building on the momentum of this legislation, the Truman Administration introduced a national mental health bill in March 1945. This legislation provided for the establishment of a national neuro-psychiatric institute (later named NIMH) and provided funds to foster research, to train mental health professionals and to provide grants-in-aid to states to establish clinics and treatment centers.

Perhaps sensitive to President Pierce's rationale for vetoing the 12,225,000 Acre Act, Felix noted [35] that the grants for mental health services did not violate the primacy of state responsibility in the care of persons with a mental illness:

> ...the primary responsibility for operating and financing services of the public health belongs to state and local communities to the limit of their resources...[but] it is the responsibility of the Public Health Service for the benefit of the whole nation to mobilize the collective knowledge of the Nation in matters pertaining to the prevention, diagnosis and treatment of illness.

Congress passed the National Mental Health Act (P.L. 79-487) in 1946. This landmark legislation established as national policy the responsibility of the federal government for the prevention and treatment of mental illness. In signing the act, President Harry S Truman reversed the action of Pierce and signaled the willingness of the federal government to share with state and local governments public responsibility for Americans with a mental illness. Exactly 100 years after Dorothea Dix petitioned for persons with a mental illness to be considered "wards of the Nation," Truman and Congress granted her wish.

In later years, Truman was to reflect that there was no single piece of health legislation approved during his term that was a source of greater pride to him than the National Mental Health Act of 1946. This president's sense of pride was well deserved. When grants to states were made available in 1948, the federal government joined state and local governments in a three-tiered intergovernmental partnership for mental health services.

The approach was extremely successful. In Truman's native Missouri, funds made available under this act, section 314 of the Public Health Service Act and later, Title V of the Health Amendments Act of 1956 (P.L. 84-911), established outreach and other outplacement clinics that were soon exclusively supported by the Missouri General Assembly. For example, in Kansas City, a few miles from Truman's home, National Mental Health Act funds helped establish a local mental health program that merited national recognition.

The Greater Kansas City Mental Health Foundation (Foundation) was formed in 1950 by progressive civic leaders in that Missouri city who wanted to upgrade the quality of mental health services for their fellow Kansas Citians[6]. Shortly after its founding, it began to administer local inpatient and outpatient treatment programs at the city's Psychiatric Receiving Center (PRC). In 1954, the Foundation was awarded a NIMH psychiatric residency training grant – a National Mental Health Act priority. In 1958, it established aftercare and day hospital programs. It also pioneered consultation and education programs through its child guidance clinic. In 1961, the Foundation was presented the *Gold Award* of the American Psychiatric Association for the excellence and com-prehensiveness of its programs and service. Two years later, its comprehensive service program was recognized as one of the eight most successful community-based mental health programs in the nation, and it was selected as a demonstration community mental health center program. Later, it would serve as the foundation for Western MO, one of the first federally funded CMHCs in America.

Similar results occurred throughout the country. Between 1946 and 1950, the number of states operating outpatient mental health services increased from 20 to 45 [35]. With state funding came new state laws dealing with the commitment of persons for mental health care, their protection and the protection of their assets by means of guardianship laws.

THE POST-WAR YEARS

In the decade immediately following the end of World War II, other forces aligned to make community-based mental health inter-ventions more feasible. They included: (1) the publication of dam-

---

[6] See the *Missouri First-Person Interview* with Dr. Robijn Hornstra [pp. 73-76] for more information on the early history of the Greater Kansas City Mental Health Foundation, its Psychiatric Receiving Center and the Western Missouri Mental Health Center.

aging critiques of life in mental institutions; (2) the emergence of coordinated and powerful mental health interest groups; (3) the introduction of effective psychopharmacology; and (4) the decentralization of public mental hospitals into geographic units.

Beginning in the late 1940s, popular periodicals such as *Reader's Digest* and *Life* magazine, as well as big city newspapers, began publishing exposés on the deplorable conditions at some public mental institutions. These reports paralleled blockbuster books such as Albert Deutsch's *The Shame of the States* [25] and Mary Jane Ward's first-person account of life in a mental institution *The Snake Pit* [109]. Equally influential were the research and writings of Alfred Stanton and Morris Schwartz, whose *The Mental Hospital* [98] reported research findings relating patient symptoms to mental hospitals' social organizations. These texts, and others like Erving Goffman's *Asylums: Essays on the Social Situation of Mental Patients and Other Inmates* [40] and *The Myth of Mental Illness* by psychiatrist Thomas Szasz [102], both published in 1961, greatly influenced the formation of mental health professionals who would soon be in the vanguard of community-based mental health care.

In 1950, the American Psychiatric Association's Psychiatric Foundation, the National Mental Health Foundation and the National Committee for Mental Hygiene joined forces to form the NMHA. Ten years later, the number of local and state voluntary mental health organizations had increased four-fold to over 800 nationwide [34]. The grassroots political clout of the NMHA would be pivotal to the passage of subsequent mental health legislation on both the national and state levels.

The year 1954 marked a watershed in the treatment of institutionalized persons suffering from psychotic disorders. In that year, reserpine, whose use dates from ancient Hindu medicine, was reintroduced as an antipsychotic agent, marking the beginning of the large-scale use of antipsychotic drugs. In the same year, the U.S. Food and Drug Administration approved the use of chlorpromazine (trade name Thorazine) for patients, after clinical trials in state mental hospitals generated stunning restorations to near-normal behaviors of patients considered incurable. The rapid and widespread use of these and related medications made possible the discharge of persons who would have otherwise been confined to such institutions for the remainder of their lives. The prospect of patient discharge raised the need for community aftercare to a new high priority, and made partial hospital programs a possibility. Furthermore, the dramatic efficacy of psychiatric medications elevated psychiatry to a more prominent position among the medical specialties, and inspired hope among professionals, patients, policymakers and the public-at-large.

Finally, administrators of large mental hospitals began to reorganize their treatment units along geographical lines. The relentless addition of new patients led to the development of a two-tier approach to patient care and patient location. Recently admitted patients were assigned to small receiving units that provided intensive diagnostic and acute treatment services. Those patients who proved to be unresponsive to acute care were relocated to wards that served persons deemed to have chronic mental illnesses – the "back wards" of state hospitals [65].

Innovators in the field began to organize hospital wards based on the geographic area from which the patients were admitted. Under this arrangement, "acute" and "chronic" patients were mixed on the same wards. Research findings by authors such as Maxwell Jones [63] on the therapeutic potential of patients on each other propelled this approach. In his writings on therapeutic communities, Jones documented that, under certain conditions, ordinary human interactions among individuals in a mental hospital setting could have more therapeutic value than professional interventions.

Social work staff from hospitals and local mental hygiene clinics created close professional linkages, accelerating hospital discharges. Teams of hospital-based professionals began to travel to the mental health and social service agencies in the areas represented on their geographic units to provide aftercare and community education.

ACTION FOR MENTAL HEALTH LEADS TO ACTION FOR MENTAL HEALTH

Despite the advances of the National Mental Health Act, the majority of persons with a mental illness continued to be treated in state and county mental hospitals. In 1955, at a point when the inpatient census in these hospitals approached 560,000 persons, Congress passed the Mental Health Study Act of 1955 (P.L. 84-142). This legislation established the Joint Commission on Mental Illness and Health (Joint Commission). Congress charged the Joint Commission to study and make recommendations on the human and economic problems of mental illness and methods for diagnosing, treating, caring for and rehabilitating persons with a mental illness. *Action for Mental Health* [62], the final report of the Joint Commission, was delivered to President Dwight D. Eisenhower on December 31, 1960, and released to the public several weeks later.

The Joint Commission proposed that the system of state mental hospitals be replaced by a comprehensive multi-institutional approach based upon:

1. Community mental health clinics for outpatient treatment
2. General hospital psychiatric units for short-term hospitalization
3. Intensive psychiatric treatment centers "for patients with major mental illnesses in the acute stages or, in the case of a more prolonged illness, those with a good prospect for improvement or recovery"
4. Chronic disease centers for long-term illnesses, including chronic mental illness.

The Joint Commission also recommended that "expenditures for public mental patient services should be doubled in the next five years – and tripled in the next ten," and that the federal government share in the cost of state and local mental health services. According to *Action for Mental Health*, "the federal government should be prepared to assume a major part of the responsibility for the mentally ill insofar as the states are agreeable to surrendering it." Three principles were to direct an expanded federal program of matching grants to the states for mental health care:

1. The federal government on the one side, and the state and local governments on the other, should share in the cost of services.

2. The total federal share should be arrived at in a series of graduated steps over a period of years, this share being determined each year on the basis of state funds spent in the previous year.

3. The grants should be awarded according to criteria of merit and incentive.

By the end of the 1950s, public pessimism over the future of persons with a mental illness was beginning to lift. The success of early psychotropic medications, generalized post-war optimism and the emergence of a push toward social equality, helped reframe persons with a mental illness as a subset of the population, worthy[7] of better living conditions and effective treatment.

THE CONCEPTION OF COMMUNITY MENTAL HEALTH CENTERS

By the 1960 election, reform of mental health care was emerging as a national political reality. Eisenhower was awaiting the final report of the Joint Commission, and the Democratic Party's platform affirmed federal support for community mental health care [89]. The Democratic president-elect, John F. Kennedy, took office as *Action for Mental Health* was being released.

Bolstered by a family interest in mental retardation specifically and mental disability issues generally, Kennedy directed Department of Health, Education and Welfare (DHEW) Secretary Anthony J. Celebrese to establish a task force to develop a response to the

---

[7] Rochefort [89] points out that the status of being "deserving" is a concept of longstanding importance in social welfare policymaking. Addresses by Royal Governor Fauquier in Virginia [p. 24] and Governor Marmaduke in Missouri [pp. 61-62], to their respective legislative bodies underscore this point, that the public will favorably consider worthwhile actions on behalf of worthy persons or causes.

Joint Commission report. The team consisted of Boisfeuillet Jones representing Celebrese; Daniel P. Moynihan representing Secretary of Labor Willard Wirtz; Felix and his deputy at NIMH, Dr. Stanley Yolles; Joint Commission economist Rashi Fein; and representatives of the Bureau of the Budget and the Veterans Administration.

Task force chairman Jones asked the NIMH leadership to prepare specific proposals to implement the Joint Commission's recommendations. In April 1962, the president's task force discussed a comprehensive community mental health centers program proposal submitted by Felix and Yolles. In the view of the NIMH chiefs, persons with a mental illness could be served better through community-based centers than through large state institutions isolated from community life. Acknowledging that there would always be a number of patients who would need institutional care, Felix and Yolles thought that over the next generation, the size of state mental hospitals could be reduced from the then current level of 525,000 patients. By 1962, Felix and NIMH had accumulated both the clinical experience in the field and the political clout in Congress to press their points. Over the period from 1948 to 1962, the annual expenditures for services, research and training at NIMH grew from $4.5 million to $106.2 million, including more than $90 million in grant funds in 1962.

The object of the task force was to eliminate the state mental hospital as it then existed[8]. The proposed substitute for the state hospital was to be the comprehensive community mental health center. The primary strategy was to minimize the state role in the provision of mental health services by making grants of federal funds to establish community mental health centers throughout the country. With these funds would come federal control in the form of regulations and standards. The NIMH proposal raised an

---

[8] During Congressional hearings on the National Mental Health Act, Felix testified: "I wish to God I could live and be active for 25 more years, because I believe if I could, I would see the day when the state mental hospitals as we know them today would no longer exist." On September 19, 1982, he participated in the dedication of a building named in his honor at the Western Missouri Mental Health Center in Kansas City's "Hospital Hill," having seen his wish come true in Missouri.

important public policy question concerning the role of state governments in developing and administering this new service network. According to Dr. Hank Foley [37]:

> Jones, Felix and Moynihan argued that it was politically and professionally inappropriate to bypass the states: politically inappropriate because such an action was counter to the pattern of then current federal-state relations; professionally inappropriate because adequate care would have to be provided in many state mental hospitals until the goal of 2,000 community mental health centers was reached...(Robert) Atwell (representing the Bureau of the Budget) argued that the states should be bypassed because they were an obstruction. Fein argued that the states were not in the position adequately to support the care of mental patients. Consequently, Fein had no objection to the position that financing mental health care should become a permanent federal subsidy.

The local-state-federal partnerships established in 1948 would be replaced by local-state and local-federal pairings. Despite these new financing arrangements, in many instances, state mental health agencies played a pivotal role in the development of CMHCs in their jurisdictions. Dr. Dick Cravens [21], Missouri Director of Community Mental Health in the early days of the federal community mental health initiative, reflected on the role each party played in Missouri in these pairings:

> State representatives, myself as a prime example, had total responsibility in consulting with communities, helping to organize local community support, reviewing and critiquing CMHC applications, indicating when the applications were ready for submission to the federal regional office in Kansas City, sitting in on the review and conferring with the review committee. Without state participation, there would have been no CMHC development at the state level ... The only time the feds consulted at the local level was when the state agency requested a consultation and that took place only with the mental

health authority present. Local people met exclusively with the state agency that administered the program.

In an effort to mollify advocates for improved state hospitals, the task force recommended several new programs[9] to upgrade the quality of services in publicly operated mental hospitals. According to Foley [37], the proposals constituted a professional and political compromise between a major effort to upgrade the care in state mental hospitals and doing nothing for the hospitals by putting all the federal resources into the CMHCs.

On February 5, 1963, President Kennedy sent a special message to Congress [64]. In it he stated,

> Mental illness and mental retardation are among our most critical health problems...Every year nearly 1,500,000 such persons receive treatment in institutions for the mentally ill and mentally retarded. Most of them are confined and compressed within an antiquated, vastly overcrowded chain of custodial institutions ... This situation has been tolerated far too long. It has troubled our national conscience – but only as a problem unpleasant to mention, easy to postpone, and despairing of solution ... The time has come for a bold new approach.

The president's "bold new approach" to mental health care was first introduced in the U.S. Senate that same month as S. 755. Congressional hearings in the Senate and House of Representatives in the late winter and spring resulted in a bill which would fund the construction and staffing of CMHCs. Opposition by the American Medical Association to what they perceived as a form of socialized medicine led to supplemental hearings in July 1963 and the

---

[9] According to Foley, the role of the states in the new federal mental health initiative was problematic. While the majority of task force members wanted to bypass the states in the administration of the CMHC program, they could make its passage difficult. Foley quotes Robert Atwell as referring to the Hospital Improvement Program (HIP) and the Hospital Staff Development (HSD) Program as a "political sop" to insure the states' endorsement of the community mental health grants.

removal of the staffing provisions in the final bill. Finally, in early fall 1963, both the House and Senate passed the bill, which was sent to President Kennedy for his signature.

Commenting on the parturition of the community mental health movement and community mental health centers, Felix [34] stated[10]:

> Thus was born the concept of the comprehensive community mental health center which was so strongly hinted at in the Joint Commission report. The feasibility of a comprehensive community mental health center was based on a number of foundation stones, without which it would have been impossible to develop the idea to the working stage. These included improvements in state mental hospitals that allowed treatment of patients in extramural settings; the advent of the psychoactive drugs; the reversal of the alarming growth of mental hospital populations; the increase in treatment of psychiatric ills in general hospitals; and the growth of the trained mental health manpower pool.

---

[10] After leaving NIMH, Dr. Felix was Dean of the St. Louis University School of Medicine. While in that post, he delivered the remarks quoted on pages 39, 41-42 and 45 in a series of lectures at Columbia University. While living in Missouri, Dr. Felix was a member of the Missouri Mental Health Commission.

2 SYSTEMS OF CARE FOR PERSONS WITH A MENTAL ILLNESS: COMMUNITY MENTAL HEALTH

PRINCIPLES OF COMMUNITY MENTAL HEALTH

Community mental health refers to organized efforts to promote and improve the mental health of a community and its members. As such, the community mental health movement's primary innovation in the practice of mental health care was contextual not clinical. Prior to the introduction of community mental health principles, the locus of activity and responsibility for the prevention and treatment of mental illness was the doctor-patient relationship. The community mental health movement shifted that locus to the CMHC-community relationship, of which the doctor-patient relationship was only one component. This innovation had its roots in the strong adherence to public health principles practiced at NIMH under Felix.[11] In lectures at Columbia University, he summarized the core concepts of community mental health:

> Whether one is talking of mental illnesses, typhoid fever, or tuberculosis, the fundamental concept is the same: the community can be nurturing and helpful or it can be toxic and hostile. In any event, if one is to recover from one's illness, whatever type it may be, one must return home

---

[11] According to Rochefort [89], in the early 1960s, "the public health viewpoint clearly dominated NIMH, which had among its employees more M.P.H. degree-holders than any other branch of the Public Health Service."

eventually. Not to do so is, in effect, not to have fully recovered. The concept of the community goes deeper than this, however, for, as with typhoid fever or tuberculosis, there can exist foci of infection which, when the circumstances are right and the patient's resistance is low, may be the producer of an illness which can incapacitate or overwhelm one. Thus, as one thinks of the rehabilitation of the individual who is already sick, one turns immediately to consideration of the factors in the community which will be supportive of the person or which will tend to be destructive. In mental illnesses and mental health, as with tuberculosis, these considerations encompass many aspects of the community. One is concerned with such problems as housing, unemployment, prejudice, and other sources of social and psychological tension in the neighborhood as well as in the home. If one is to carry this concept to its logical conclusion, one would say that a community can be therapeutic or destructive, depending upon a variety of elements. By therapeutic is meant supportive and helpful in all aspects, not merely through the organized agencies whose responsibility is caretaking. When these factors exist in a community and there is added the element of skilled personnel to care for those who need professional help, the community contains within itself the elements necessary to maintain or restore health, mental or physical. By the same token, as one considers those who are not yet overtly ill but who are vulnerable, the same elements in the community are important. Appropriate facilities for emotional support, when needed, and for advice and counseling, when indicated, can spell the difference between continued health and mental illness. Finally, the positive aspects of mental health must be given attention. Within the community should lie those factors for character building and for positive mental health which contribute to a more rugged and resilient state of mental health. This means much more than merely fending off mental illness.

In practice, this philosophy was carried out through the following eight principles.

Responsibility for a specified population

Under the federal CMHC program, state agencies designated as State Mental Health Authorities were required to divide their jurisdictions into catchment areas[12] of 75,000 to 200,000 persons each. According to Foley [37], this number was arrived at on the spur of the moment by Felix. When asked about the optimal size of a catchment area, he simply divided the president's task force's projected need for 2,000 CMHCs into a population base of 200 million persons. Further massaging of this estimate created a range with the low end judged large enough to be cost effective and the high end small enough to be manageable.

The ensuing debates about the relevance of the population approach to defining a community, especially in light of more appropriate sociological definitions[13], have often clouded the critical aspect of designating catchment areas: assigning responsibility for the promotion of mental health and the treatment and rehabilitation of mental illness for all persons in a specific geographic area. Under the provisions of each state's mental health plan, the mental health and illness needs of all of its citizens, and thereby all Americans, would be assigned to and become the responsibility of a qualified mental health agency, whether public or private. In today's parlance, responsibility for a specified population would guarantee that the needs of un-served and under-served groups in a specified geographic area would be addressed in a comprehensive manner by a qualified mental health organization.

---

[12] The use of the term *catchment area* to define the service area of a CMHC is one of many examples of the influence of the public health ideology of the early framers of CMHC policy and practice. In this text, the terms *catchment area* and *service area* are used interchangeably.

[13] For example, Register [88] enumerates 11.

43

Focus on prevention and early intervention

Early framers of the CMHC ideology recognized that at the local, state and federal levels there were likely insufficient funds to pay, in perpetuity, for the treatment and rehabilitation of persons with a mental illness or serious emotional disturbance. For the public health oriented policymakers at NIMH, a partial solution to this problem was the practice of primary and secondary prevention. Simply stated, in mental health[14]:

> *Primary prevention* refers to the reduction in the incidence, or number of new cases, of mental illness by identifying and minimizing its causes.

> *Secondary prevention* refers to the reduction in the prevalence, or total number of cases, of mental illness through early identification and prompt, effective treatment.

> *Tertiary prevention* refers to the reduction in the handicapping effects of a mental illness through rehabilitation and case management.

CMHC grant recipients were required to provide consultation and education services, a popular form of primary prevention. Although these services were not reimbursed through the CMHC grant process until 1975, books and training on mental health consultation quickly abounded. By 1975, senior NIMH administrators [71] were able to publish a catalogue of 1,136 books, journal and periodical articles, tapes and videos on mental health consultation, spanning the country from Dr. Meiji Singh [95] in Berkeley to Dr. Gerald Caplan[15] [12, 13, 14, 15] in Boston.

---

[14] Some mental health professionals add a fourth, or *quaternary* level of prevention, which refers to the reduction in the handicapping effects of participating in a human management system through advocacy and staff development.

[15] Dr. Caplan's impact on the community mental health movement cannot be overstated. In addition to his prolific writing on primary prevention, especially mental health consultation, he also established and directed the Laboratory of Community Psychiatry at Harvard Medical School, a training ground for many leaders in the CMHC movement at the federal, state and center levels.

Treating people with a mental illness in their home communities

This principle, stated repeatedly in President Kennedy's Message to Congress and in Congressional testimony by NIMH officials, mental health advocates and professional supporters of the CMHC Act, is the clearest objective of the CMHC movement. Proponents of CMHC development reference it as the fulfillment of the vision set forth in *Action for Mental Health,* and the solution to the problem of inadequate care in public mental hospitals. Felix [34] directly addressed this issue, set in the context of prevention:

> This whole problem of patient population as it relates to public mental hospitals, with all it connotes in terms of treatment procedures, staffing patterns, employee morale, and the like, had been a matter of concern to those working in the mental health field for many years. Somehow it did not seem that hospitalization in large institutions, sometimes far removed from the homes of the patients, was a logical procedure. If one were to relate procedures and treatments to the etiology of illness it seemed as though more attention should be given to keeping the patient in his home community. This concept centered on the fact that people who become mentally ill usually become so in their homes, among their family members, in their own neighborhoods. Their illness is not an isolated occurrence, dependent on nothing around them. If they become ill in the community, if the community is in truth a contributing factor in their illness, then it must follow that true recovery, or even recovery to such an extent that they can function effectively hinges upon adjustment to and in the community. By community is meant home, work, and neighborhood. This belief encompasses a number of medical and psychiatric concepts including a public health approach to the problem, the primary idea of which is prevention.

Research by Drs. Elaine and John Cumming[16] [23], documenting the adverse effects on later re-entry of removing persons with a mental illness from their home communities, helped provide a strong rationale for this principle.

Provision of a continuum of care

The community mental health ideology considers the principle of *continuum of care* from two perspectives. From one perspective, it refers to the federal requirement that CMHC grantees provide a comprehensive program of mental health and mental illness services for all persons in their respective catchment areas. At first, this continuum of direct services included emergency, inpatient, outpatient and partial hospitalization services. In 1975, Congress added the requirement for special services for children and the elderly, transitional services and follow-up care for discharged patients, pre-admission screening for persons being considered for admission into a public mental hospital, and alcohol and drug abuse services.

From the other perspective, the principle of *continuum of care* refers to the commitment to do whatever is necessary so that individual consumers can be retained in their home communities and maintain productive lives there. This second meaning gained additional value as CMHCs began to provide services to persons with mental illnesses that were more severe and persistent.

Use of multidisciplinary teams, including paraprofessional staff

A major thrust of the National Mental Health Act was the preparation of mental health professionals across a broad spectrum of disciplines: psychiatry, psychology, social work and nursing. Prepared to function in multidisciplinary teams, these mental health professionals were encouraged to include among their ranks

---

[16] Dr. John Cumming would later serve on the staff of the Kansas City Mental Health Foundation.

paraprofessional staff, many drawn from the membership of the local community, some former clients. The addition of paraprofessionals had many positive effects on CMHC operations, both in the quality of care provided and in community acceptance. For example, Stuart Golann and Carl Eisdorfer [41] pointed out that indigenous persons providing services also helped "bridge the gap between psychodynamically oriented socially advantaged mental health professionals and disadvantaged clients concerned with the effects of bigotry, poverty and powerlessness."

Linkages with other community organizations and agencies

CMHCs have long been characterized by two prominent features: (1) a lack of sufficient funds to address all of the mental health needs in their respective communities; and (2) an interest in collaborating with other community agencies for early intervention, referral and community support. Since their origins in the child guidance movement, community-based clinicians have worked collaboratively with schools, child welfare agencies and other social service organizations dealing with children and families. Linkages with organizations as diverse as correctional institutions and "Main Street" employers have proven beneficial to enterprising CMHCs, both financially and from a public relations point of view. The proliferation of smaller mental health related agencies (e.g., rape crisis centers) and the emergence of influential consumer and family advocacy groups have added to the number of opportunities for linkage by CMHCs.

Fiscal and program accountability

The initial CMHC legislation and its early amendments were passed in an era of major social reform legislation that empowered many smaller, community-oriented and not-for-profit welfare, health and educationally oriented organizations to bring about improvements in the lives of individuals at local levels. Incorporated in this legislation were firm requirements for fiscal reporting and the measurement of program outcomes. In the mental health arena, the field of program evaluation blossomed, a major role being played by psychologists. Publications by NIMH [51] and prominent researchers in the field [94, 112] spawned a wide range of evaluation specialists and studies. Throughout the 1970s, regional associations of state programs such as the Southern Regional Education Board, the Western Interstate Commission for Higher Education, and the National Association of State Mental Health Program Directors (NASMHPD) routinely coordinated technical training for program evaluators in the mental health field.

Citizen participation

Although passed in the era of federal legislation promoting social reform and citizen empowerment at the local level,[17] in the beginning of the federal CMHC program, there was no require-ment that a center's board of directors include citizens who were not mental health professionals, or that it be broadly represen-tative of the backgrounds and interests of community members. Nevertheless, private citizens were often the driving force in seeking federal funds. According to Cravens [20],

> In these early days, the community decision makers were comfortable in identifying a local problem, then organ-izing to form an incorporated board or identifying an existing body to pursue the federal CMHC dollar. This nucleus group was not necessarily representative of the community to be served. Racial and ethnic minorities were not present; neither were women, unless they were physicians or elected officials; and likewise the poor were left out of the picture. If planning took place in a rural setting, the farmer was a member only if he were wealthy or happened to be an elected official.

---

[17] For example, the Economic Opportunity Act of 1964 required that anti-poverty programs be designed and implemented with the *maximum feasible participation* of those served. See Moynihan [81] for an analysis of this legislative term.

By 1971, NIMH [84] published regulations that required broader community participation in this form:

> Community mental health centers must involve the community in the planning, development and operation of the program ... the participating citizens must include board representation of all elements of the community such as professionals, lay persons, appropriate consumers, persons from the range of socioeconomic groups, cultural groups, age groups (youth, adults and aged) and geographic and political subdivisions.

COMMUNITY MENTAL HEALTH LEGISLATION 1963-1980

On October 31, 1963, President John F. Kennedy signed into law the Mental Retardation and Community Mental Health Centers Act of 1963. Title II of this act, referred to as the Community Mental Health Centers Act (CMHC Act) made grants, ranging from 66⅔% to 33⅓% for the construction of community mental health centers, patterned after the highly successful Hill-Burton program[18] for planning and constructing hospitals.

Centers that received funds were required to develop a service delivery system for their communities that: (1) was responsive to current community mental illness treatment needs; (2) promoted positive mental health for individuals at risk of developing a mental illness; and (3) was integrated with other mental health services in and for their communities. These services were expected to be geographically, culturally and linguistically accessible, and financially affordable to all segments of the community, and to provide for a continuum of care. At a minimum, the service array was required to include five *essential services*: inpatient, outpatient, partial hospitalization service, 24-hour emergency, and consultation and education services for community agencies and professional personnel. CMHC Act grantees agreed to provide these services for 20 years.

---

[18] Hospital Survey and Construction Act of 1946 (P.L. 79-725).

Two years later, the Community Mental Health Amendments of 1965 reinstated staffing provisions first planned for the 1963 act. These original staffing grants were for a period of 51 months with a declining federal investment from 75% in the first 15 months to 30% for the final year. The Mental Health Amendments of 1967 (P.L. 90-31) extended the construction and staffing grants for another three years, supplying sufficient funds to pay for the nearly 300 CMHCs then established and approximately 300 new centers. Later, Congress re-authorized the CMHC legislation for another three years, extending the length of staffing grants to eight years, adding funds for children's mental health services and consultation and education services, as well as providing more favorable match levels for CMHCs operating in federally designated poverty areas. In 1973, Congress provided for a one-year extension included in the Health Programs Extension Act of 1973 (P.L. 93-245).

The Community Mental Health Amendments of 1975 (P.L. 94-63) extended and expanded the CMHC Act for another two years, adding this preamble:

> The Congress finds that (1) community mental health care is the most effective and humane form of care for a majority of mentally ill individuals; (2) the federally funded community mental health centers have had a major impact on the improvement of mental health care ... and thus are a national resource to which all Americans should enjoy access; and (3) there is currently a shortage of quality community mental health care resources in the United States.
>
> The Congress further declares that federal funds should continue to be made available for the purposes of initiating new and continuing existing community mental health centers and initiating new services within centers, and for the monitoring of the performance of all federally funded centers to insure their responsiveness to community needs and national goals relating to community mental health care.

This act introduced major changes in the basic CMHC program, including the addition of seven new essential services to the original five. The new services targeted children, the elderly, and persons with drug and alcohol problems; and they required pre-admission screening for persons believed to require public mental hospital care and transitional and follow-up care for persons discharged from inpatient mental health care.

When former Georgia Governor Jimmy Carter succeeded President Gerald Ford in 1977, community mental health supporters gained proven champions of humane, effective community-based mental health care in the new president and his first lady, Rosalynn. Early in his administration, Carter signaled his intense interest in advancing the community mental health agenda by establishing the President's Commission on Mental Health, with his wife as Honorary Chairperson. Established on February 17, 1977, the President's Commission was charged with reviewing the mental health needs of the United States and making recommendations as to how best serve these needs. Commission members held hearings around the country and established 35 task panels to conduct in-depth studies and to make recommendations on critical questions.

The President's Commission generated public and professional enthusiasm and many suggested improvements. One set of improvements dealt with the extension of the Medicaid intermediate care facilities program to provide funding for persons with a mental illness. At its inception, Medicaid was made unavailable as a revenue source for services to persons between the ages of 22 and 64 in healthcare facilities referred to as "institutions for mental diseases," code for mental hospitals. Ironically, the availability of Medicaid funding for institutional, and later, community-based intermediate care programs for persons with mental retardation and other developmental disabilities was a major force in the elimination of substandard treatment in these settings. Advocates for persons with a mental illness were eager for similar benefits to apply for persons hospitalized with these disabilities.

Another suggested innovation redefined the relationships among local, state and federal agencies in the continued expansion of the community mental health centers program, enhancing the role of the state mental health authority in planning and monitoring the distribution of federal CMHC funds in their states. By mid-1980, the number of CMHCs had grown to over 750, covering half the nation and serving 105 million persons. The total federal investment had been $2.29 billion [93], which was supplemented by a combined state investment of $4.5 billion [19]. At that time, the centers received approximately $320 million annually from NIMH and $400 million from state governments. However, these federal funds constituted only a small portion of the mental disabilities funding made available by the federal government[19]. Even the state share of CMHC operations was a small portion of its total mental health funding effort.

These changes, and an expanded CMHC grant program, were embodied in the Mental Health Systems Act of 1980 (P.L. 96-398). When this legislation was signed by President Carter on October 7, 1980, mental health advocates believed that their long push for continuity in the CMHC program was finally within reach. Their optimism was short-lived. The advances represented in this act were undone by the Reagan Administration, which took office less than four months after it was signed into law. Through the Omnibus Budget Reconciliation Act of 1981 (OBRA, P.L. 97-35), the administration collapsed 57 federal categorical aid programs[20] into nine block grants[21]. One of these, the alcohol, drug abuse and

---

[19] For example, in FY 1979, only $1.02 billion (12.67%) of the $8.039 billion of Department of Health, Education and Welfare expenditures were distributed through the Alcohol, Drug Abuse and Mental Health Administration (then home of the NIMH) and the Developmental Disabilities Office [93].

[20] By the start of the Reagan Administration, there were approximately 600 categorical grants to state and local governments.

[21] The Advisory Commission on Intergovernmental Relations [1] has defined a block grant as "a program by which funds are provided chiefly to general purpose government units in accordance with a statutory formula for use in a broad functional area, largely at the recipient's discretion." First employed by the Johnson Administration in 1966, by 1974 the Nixon and Ford Administrations had brought the total number of block grants to five.

mental health services (ADAMH) block grant lumped together ten categorical and project grant-in-aid programs. Grant requirements were reduced, but so were total federal funds, by approximately one-fourth. These changes effectively closed out expansion of the federal community mental health centers program.

The ADAMH block grant limited states' discretion in the early years. In the first year of the grant (federal fiscal year 1982), states were required to replicate the balance of federal mental health and substance abuse funding that was operative in the prior year. In succeeding years, small variations in prior funding patterns were permitted. In time, the "block" feature of these grants was eroded by the passage of quasi-categorical funding, especially in the area of anti-drug abuse initiatives. In practice, few of these new funds were made available for community mental health services.

The original OBRA legislation and its re-authorizing legislation required states to continue funding all federally initiated community mental health centers that received federal CMHC funding in federal fiscal year 1981, and that would have been eligible for continued funding in the current fiscal year. In order to receive funds through the ADAMH block grant, participating CMHCs were expected to provide a comprehensive array of services, regardless of a consumer's ability to pay. The recommended service array included outpatient, day treatment/partial hospitalization, 24-hour emergency services, consultation and education, and pre-admission screening for persons seeking admission to a state mental hospital. States had broad latitude in determining the level of block grant funds provided to individual centers, as long as all eligible centers received block grant support.

The pattern of adding categorical "set-asides" in the ADAMH block grant took its toll on states' discretion in funding community mental health services. For example, the 1988 amendments to the block grant program required states to spend at least 55% of their mental health allocation to fund new mental health programs. Earlier amendments had required that 10% of mental health block grant funds be set aside for various underserved populations, especially severely emotionally disturbed youth.

SOCIAL SECURITY REFORM AND THE REDISTRIBUTION OF INPATIENT CARE

At the same time as the community mental health centers concept was being developed, the Social Security system was changing in ways that were compatible with the community mental health agenda. Beginning in 1960, the Social Security Act was amended to allow up to six weeks of care in a public mental hospital for certain persons who were elderly and indigent. In 1962, federal DHEW regulations were revised to permit welfare payments for persons on conditional release from public mental hospitals [89].

The changes in health care coverage brought about by the passage of the Title XVIII (Medicare) and Title XIX (Medicaid) Amendments to the Social Security Act in 1965 had a prominent impact on services for persons with a mental illness. Both Medicare and Medicaid permitted the use of federal assistance for the treatment of eligible elderly persons in psychiatric hospitals[22]. Medicare set a lifetime limit of 190 days for reimbursed treatment in a mental institution, with no limitation for care provided in general hospitals [44]. These changes both improved the quality of care for elderly persons in state hospitals and promoted the transfer of others to general hospitals and nursing homes, which were eager to accept both the patients and their available federal reimbursements.

Happily for community mental health proponents, both Medicare and Medicaid placed no restrictions on reimbursements for treatment provided to eligible consumers in general hospitals. At this time, community hospitals were being encouraged either to submit a federal CMHC grant application or to provide the inpatient services needed by another community applicant. The availability of federal reimbursement for inpatient care was a tremendous incentive to establish these services which, in the words of Kennedy, "make it possible for most of the mentally ill to be successfully and quickly treated in their own communities and returned to a useful place in society."

---

[22] Medicaid specifically excluded reimbursement for persons under age 65 in "institutions for mental diseases."

Summarizing the impact of amendments to federal "welfare" legislation Grob [44] notes that:

> Whatever the reasons, there is little doubt that mental hospitals had changed dramatically by the 1970s ... Between 1970 and 1982 the average number of patients per employee fell from 1.7 to 0.7, as compared with 6.8 in 1945, 3.83 in 1955 and 2.42 in 1965. By 1980, the median stay in public institutions was 23 days, although sharp differences for specific diagnoses existed (for alcohol- and drug-related conditions the median stay was 12 days, for organic disorders 71, for affective disorders 22, and for schizophrenia 42). That public hospitals remained a place of last resort for certain chronic and severely mentally ill patients is evident from the fact that the mean length-of-stay in 1980 was 165 days.

These effects were predicted by Felix in 1963 [32] when he forecast the effect of CMHC development on state mental hospitals:

> All of this will, of course, have a tremendous impact on the state mental hospitals as we know them today. It should be apparent that these hospitals will not be eliminated in the foreseeable future, though they will no longer be the sole treatment resource available to the general population of any particular community.
>
> Far from being eliminated, this program, when fully implemented, will make it possible for the mental hospital to function as an effective and essential resource for specialized groups of patients within a comprehensive program of mental health care....The treatment such patients will receive in the future will be active and intensive. They will not be shunted aside to be ignored and forgotten. The hospital will, for these patients, regain a meaning that is now lost to many of them.

Later [33], he elaborated on his vision of the future of public mental hospitals:

...as the public mental hospitals are relieved of responsibility to treat thousands of patients who should not be hospitalized there ... they can improve services to those who do need hospitalization. And they can also expand the services which will make the hospital an integral part of the entire community-based treatment program.

THE SHIFT TO SERVICES FOR PERSONS WITH SERIOUS AND PERSISTENT MENTAL ILLNESSES

In its original form, the legislation that eventually became the Mental Health Systems Act of 1980 provided for a limited number of demonstration projects whereby federally selected state mental health agencies would manage the federal community mental health center funds in their jurisdictions. This approach proved to be problematic for state mental health agency directors since federal CMHC funds constituted a small fraction of total mental health expenditures managed by their agencies.[23]   In 1979, NASMHPD, led by the mental health directors in Maine and Missouri, drafted a substitute for DHEW's Mental Health Systems Act proposals. NASMHPD's substitute bill, the Partnership for Mental Health Act of 1979, proposed a mechanism whereby any state mental health authority that could meet federal criteria would be eligible through a performance contract process to administer federal CMHC funds as an *exclusive contractor* for NIMH [2]. This provision was eventually incorporated in the final version of the Mental Health Systems Act.

Even though this act was never implemented, the exercise of developing alternate bill language provided a focal point for state mental health directors to develop strategies and procedures for managing future federal CMHC funds. This period of rehearsal

---

[23] State governments spent $2.2 billion more than the federal government on the community mental health centers program during the first 13 years of its history [19], and by 1980, states spent nine dollars for every federal dollar spent on mental health [18].

proved in most instances to be beneficial both to the state mental health agencies and to the community mental health centers in their jurisdictions, when the federal block grants were substituted for categorical grants.

The state-community pairing gave state agencies additional leverage to address an area of burgeoning professional concern and public outcry: meeting the needs of persons with serious and persistent mental illnesses in the community. The emergence of the National Alliance for the Mentally Ill (NAMI) in the early 1980s added a powerful counterweight to established advocacy efforts promoting the robust agenda of the community mental health movement. These forces were also strongly felt at the federal level, where several initiatives on behalf of persons with serious and persistent mental illness were rolled out to the states. Among these were NIMH's Community Support Program in 1977 and National Plan for the Chronically Mentally Ill in 1980. The State Comprehensive Mental Health Services Plan Act of 1986 (P.L. 99-660), which was re-authorized under the Mental Health Amendments of 1990 (P.L. 101-639), required states to develop plans with a special focus on persons with serious and persistent mental illnesses.

Finally, early and mid-1980s budget crises in many states forced their mental health agencies to target funding of community-based services toward persons with a serious and persistent mental illness, especially those who had been discharged from state mental hospitals or would otherwise have been admitted there. By the late 1980s, CMHCs were less dependent on federal block grants funds as a percent of their revenues. One factor that contributed to that outcome was the expansion of Medicaid-reimbursed services provided by CMHCs. According to Jerrell and Larsen [59, 60, 61], other common strategies to adjust to the new fiscal realities facing CMHCs were increases in productivity, cutting back on service locations, and consolidating staffing[24].

---

[24] A similar response to shifts in funding was described by Naierman, Haskins and Robinson [83] in their 1978 study of CMHCs graduating from federal financial support.

Policy and funding shifts began to take their toll on the comprehensive program first envisioned for CMHCs. Whereas at their inception CMHCs were proposed as agencies specializing in primary and secondary prevention (i.e., mental health promotion and prompt, effective treatment for emerging mental health disorders), 20 years later they were functioning at the secondary and tertiary levels of prevention (treatment and rehabilitation), especially for persons with a serious and persistent mental illness. Rochefort [89] has summarized the research of Jerrell and Larsen [59, 60, 61] on these nationwide service shifts as follows:

> Although some types of CMHC services have grown in volume, others have shrunk, most notably consultation and education, prevention, and alcohol and drug treatment[25].... These services, formerly required of centers by the federal government, do not represent current priorities for state mental health authorities, nor are they usually income generating. Centers have found it possible, however, to reorient selected other services...For example, outpatient care increasingly has been redirected to two quite different, sometimes physically separated, clientele groups: chronic patients (e.g., for medication and for crisis visits) and privately paying patients.

CMHCs in many states, including Missouri, also worked to maintain a balanced program of services for a broad array of consumers by increasing fund raising in their home areas. Where appropriate, they applied the CMHC philosophy to new, high-priority service recipients. Paradoxically, dedication to these principles (e.g., responsibility for a defined population) later led some states and centers to embrace the Trojan Horse of for-profit managed behavioral health care, in some cases jeopardizing the preservation of their principles, the well-being of their consumers and the viability of their agencies.

---

[25] Contrary to this national trend, the preponderance of the 22 CMHCs in Missouri provide services to persons with a drug or alcohol problem.

PART II: COMMUNITY MENTAL HEALTH IN MISSOURI

For more than 150 years, the people of Missouri have cared for their neighbors with mental illnesses and serious emotional disorders. The next four chapters chronicle this history of caring from the establishment of the first public mental hospital west of the Mississippi River, through the active years of state and private CMHC expansion, to the consolidation of recent years. Like their counterparts in other states, mental health programs in Missouri have adjusted to wide swings in funding availability, both federal and state, and have prevailed. In 2003, DMH and its CMHC partners are well positioned to use prudently new investments of state funds whenever economic prosperity returns to Missouri.

Chapter 3 documents the expansion of mental health services in Missouri, first through the development of state-operated mental hospitals, and later as a pioneer in the arena of community mental health. Key actors in the early days of the state of Missouri's CMHC program share their reflections in their *Missouri First-Person Interviews*.

Chapter 4 details the history of private, not-for-profit mental health centers, both federally funded and not, in Missouri. When the DMH state plan for community mental health centers was first devised, 3 of the 36 catchment areas were served by state-operated CMHCs. Revisions to these catchment area boundaries in 1982 and 1997 have reduced that number to 25. The stories of 19 centers that serve 21 of these areas unfold in this chapter. The reflections of persons involved in the development of private CMHCs in Missouri are captured in their *Missouri First-Person Interviews*.

The early 1980s brought marked changes in the relationship between DMH and Missouri CMHCs, including the privatization of the state-operated CMHCs. These changes are discussed in Chapter 5, with *Missouri First-Person Interviews* featuring CMHC CEOs and key DMH staff.

Finally, Chapter 6 considers the current state of the eight principles of the community mental health movement, and details ways in which CMHCs have adapted to changing circumstances. Current CMHC CEOs join in a discussion of ongoing issues confronting the mental health system in Missouri.

3 STATE MENTAL HOSPITALS TO STATE COMMUNITY MENTAL HEALTH CENTERS (1851 TO 1966)

EARLY SERVICES FOR PERSONS WITH A MENTAL ILLNESS

In 1835, the Missouri General Assembly had made the care of insane persons the responsibility of counties[26] [22]. In some cases, guardians were appointed to care for these persons; in other cases they were provided for in county poorhouses. The first public mental hospital west of the Mississippi River was opened in Fulton, Missouri, in 1851. The availability of a specialized facility was a great improvement over both of these approaches for dealing with Missouri's mentally disordered citizens.

The first call for a hospital to treat insane persons came in November 1844 from Governor Miles Marmaduke, the eighth governor of Missouri. Nine months earlier, Governor Marmaduke succeeded Governor Thomas Reynolds, who had committed suicide. According to Dr. Hank Guhleman [46], the newspapers reported the death as "an act of insanity." In his message to the Missouri General Assembly, itself faintly reminiscent of Royal Governor Fauquier's remarks 78 years earlier to the Virginia House of Burgesses, the governor stated [46]: "We must treat these miserable beings...as fit subjects for our compassion and not

---

[26] More than 150 years later, Missouri counties would begin to tax themselves to provide for local services for persons with a mental illness following the passage of SB 168 by the 75th General Assembly in 1969.

objects of punishment." Early support stalled, but was revived in 1847, coincident with the presence in Missouri of Dorothea Dix.[27] Closed temporarily during the "War Between the States," at which time it was exploited by Union and Confederate troops alike, Fulton State Hospital has been in continuous operation since 1863.

Difficulties in transporting patients across the Missouri River to Fulton led St. Louis County, then not connected to St. Charles by a bridge, to establish its own asylum in 1869.[28] After the separation of St. Louis City and County in 1875 it was transferred to city control. State mental hospitals followed in St. Joseph (1874), Nevada (1887) and Farmington (1903), completing what Crighton [22] referred to as "Missouri's plan for the care of its insane":

> ...to provide in each of the four corners of the state a mental hospital; in addition, there was the Fulton hospital in the center of the state.

In 1948, the St. Louis City Sanitarium was transferred to the state of Missouri for one dollar. Little else changed in the first half of the 20th century, except for progressive overcrowding in state mental hospitals. In the two decades between 1920 and 1940, the institutionalized population at Missouri state mental hospitals grew at a rate seven to eight times the rate of growth of the general population. In 1947, a comprehensive study of conditions in these hospitals commissioned by the Missouri House of Representatives

---

[27] Dr. Guhleman [46] notes that, during the 14th General Assembly in 1847, "Dorothea Dix...was in St. Louis. Her influence, if any, seems to have been behind the scenes in this case, as neither the legislative journals nor newspapers mention her direct participation." However, according to Fulton State Hospital records [48], Ms. Dix visited the hospital in 1859, and generated considerable monetary donations.

[28] The order of St. Vincent de Paul, came to St. Louis in 1845 and established the St. Vincent Insane Asylum at the corner of Marion and Decatur shortly thereafter. At the time of the opening of the St. Louis County Lunatic Asylum, St. Vincent's housed 149 inmates, about one-fifth of whom were charity cases. [92]. In 1896, the asylum was moved to a site just outside the city limits of Normandy (near the current University of Missouri -St. Louis campus), where, at 500 beds, it was, according to Crighton [22], "the largest and possibly the finest asylum in the United States."

documented that only 5.4% of the patients were receiving active treatment. This report also pointed out the desperate shortage of mental health professional staff at state mental facilities [78].

Overcrowding and inadequate staffing were not reserved to state hospitals in Missouri. In the early 1930s, St. Louis general practitioner Dr. Malcolm A. Bliss successfully promoted support for a separate psychiatric unit in that city's hospital program. In 1938, the Malcolm Bliss Psychopathic Hospital was opened with a capacity of approximately 200 inpatients [104]. When a research team headed by Washington University's Dr. George Ulett came aboard in 1953, just 15 years later, he found [106]:

> a hospital that was 100 percent overcrowded, with insufficient budget, unpainted buildings, patients in restraints and without full-time psychiatrists.

According to Guhleman [45],[29] Missouri in the 1950s was:

> a mental health desert. There were oases of mental health activities scattered throughout the state, but isolated as each group or service was working alone on its own.

Dr. Milton Fujita [39], former superintendent of St. Louis State Hospital, recalled his first experience there in 1959, as a junior year medical student at St. Louis University Medical School:

> There were over a thousand patients there; they were wall-to-wall. Each of us was assigned four or five patients, and for each patient we had to write a yearly progress note for the record. Once a year: that's how bad it was. They did one follow-up progress note a year by medical students; they didn't have enough staff. When I went back as superintendent in 1980, there were 650 patients, and that was crowded. There were nearly twice that number in 1959.

---

[29] See also the *Missouri First-Person Interview* with Dr. Guhleman [pp. 69-72].

ORIGINS OF COMMUNITY-BASED MENTAL HEALTH CARE

By the early 1950s, there were small teacher training programs in St. Louis City and fledgling child guidance clinics in St. Louis County and St. Joseph. In Kansas City, civic-minded philanthropists were beginning to make plans for the establishment of the PRC. In 1952, the Division of Mental Diseases began to make grants to community groups to establish mental health clinics, as well as to state hospitals to expand their aftercare services into communities. These grants were made available through federal 314 (d) funds, which were authorized by Section 314 of the Public Health Service Act of 1944. That act revised and consolidated all of the prior legislation dealing with the Public Health Service. Section 314 of Part B (Federal-State Cooperation) dealt with grants to the states for public health services. Initially dealing with venereal disease and tuberculosis control and the establishment of local health departments, through its amendments this act became the basis for most federal-state public health initiatives. Section 314 (d) required that 15% of the funds distributed under this section be used for mental health services. In Missouri, the mental health share was $50,000 for the first year, with annual increases of $10,000 [45]. Placement of these early federal grants in the context of the Public Health Service Act demonstrates the extent to which federal health policymakers viewed mental illness as a serious public health concern.

Recently, Guhleman [45] observed that:

> By 1955, the General Assembly enacted a bill requiring the establishment of six "traveling clinics" with these services to be provided mainly in rural areas. An interesting aspect of this legislative mandate is that a number of these "traveling clinics" later became the nucleus for the establishment of community mental health centers.

These traveling clinics were staffed by teams of mental health professionals (psychiatrists, psychologists, social workers and other therapists) who worked primarily with discharged patients in their home communities. Crighton [22] provides a summary of the scope of the traveling clinics as follows:

> Farmington State Hospital was a pioneer in the development of traveling clinics and served Cape Girardeau, Dexter and Marble Hill. Fulton dispatched traveling teams to Hermann, Hannibal and Rolla. St. Louis State Hospital held clinics in Jefferson, Pike, Franklin and Lincoln counties.

In 1957, the Missouri General Assembly passed sweeping legislation that would serve to catapult Missouri's mental health system to the forefront of the states within ten years. Spearheaded by Senator Albert Spradling and House Majority Floor Leader (and future governor) Warren E. Hearnes, and a key component of Governor James T. Blair's agenda, this legislation created an independent mental health commission and established the position of executive director of the Division of Mental Diseases. The commission's selection to fill this post was Addison M. Duval, M.D., then assistant superintendent of St. Elizabeths Hospital in Washington, D.C., and a nationally prominent psychiatrist [47]. Duval got to work developing a ten-year plan for mental health.

Released in 1960, Duval's plan proposed upgrading the staffing and physical plants at the state's five mental hospitals, releasing patients to nursing and boarding facilities, subsidizing psychiatric care in general hospitals, establishing community treatment centers and expanding outpatient services. The plan was universally applauded by professional and advocacy groups and adopted by recently inaugurated Governor John Dalton, who incorporated its recommendations for improving hospital facilities in his first budget requests. However, differences between Duval and Dalton surfaced, and by November 30, 1961, the doctor was out.

Shortly thereafter, George A. Ulett, M.D., a Washington University professor of psychiatry and medical director at Malcolm Bliss Mental Health Center in St. Louis, was offered the post of director of the Division of Mental Hygiene. First agreeing to take the position on an acting basis, Ulett ultimately accepted a permanent appointment, asserting his commitment to professional training and research as a means to improve the quality of mental health care[30].

REGIONAL INTENSIVE TREATMENT CENTERS

In April 1962, Ulett unveiled a plan for the establishment of three intensive treatment centers at Malcolm Bliss in St. Louis, the PRC in Kansas City and a proposed new facility to be co-located with the University of Missouri Medical School in Columbia. According to the Executive Committee for Mental Health Planning, [30], these centers, scheduled to open in 1966, would be comprehensive in nature, providing the full range of community mental health care, including:

1. Outpatient and inpatient service for adults and children
2. Partial hospitalization services, such as day care, night care, and weekend care
3. Emergency services available 24 hours a day
4. Diagnostic services
5. Teaching
6. Rehabilitation
7. Special services for children, alcoholics and the aged
8. Research
9. Consultation and education
10. Aftercare

This plan was presented to the Missouri General Assembly in 1963 and was approved. According to Ulett [105],

> A new federal law, P.L. 88-164, had just made federal funds available on a matching basis for the creation of community mental health facilities. This new law had been anticipated by Missouri's planners.

---

[30] See Dr. Ulett's *Missouri First-Person Interview* [pp. 77-82].

In fact, as the history of the growth of the Greater Kansas City Mental Health Foundation's services at the PRC documents[1], these services already were part of the Kansas City program and were being offered at the revitalized Malcolm Bliss in St. Louis. When Mid-MO was opened, it completed the plan for intensive treatment centers and pioneered community mental health services nationwide as well as in its predominantly rural catchment area of Boone, Carroll, Chariton, Cooper, Howard, Moniteau, Morgan, Pettis, Randolph and Saline counties.

In the decade between 1957 and 1967, Missouri made significant gains in the area of community-based mental health services. In 1965, a proven advocate for the mentally ill, Warren E. Hearnes, was inaugurated governor of Missouri[2]. Recognizing that Missouri had finally "abandoned its role of laggert in its program for treatment of the mentally ill and mentally retarded," Hearnes [107] stated that "the problems of the mentally ill are age old but there are solutions and even though these solutions are not immediate, they must be our goals." Ulett [107] summarized these goals:

> Governor Hearnes recommended the establishment and support of nine regional diagnostic and treatment centers for the mentally retarded; that maximum financial support be given for the three intensive treatment centers for the mentally ill that had been authorized by the 72nd General Assembly which were established in St. Louis, Columbia, and Kansas City; and that more attention be given to salaries received by the workers in the state program. These goals reached fruition during Governor Hearnes' tenure.

In 1966, the authors of *Comprehensive Mental Health Planning in Missouri* [30] summarized the past, present and future of Missouri mental health as follows:

---

[1] See the *Missouri First-Person Interviews* with Dr. Robijn Hornstra [pp. 73-76].

[2] See the *Missouri First-Person Interviews* with Governor Warren E. Hearnes and his wife, Representative Betty Cooper Hearnes [pp. 83-86].

That an ignoble history does not necessarily portent an inglorious future is evidenced by the fact that Missouri has made greater progress in terms of mental health in the past eight years – and especially the past four years – than it did in all of its first 106 years, since the establishment of its first mental hospital in Fulton in 1851.

Missouri, then, is in an excellent position to move forward with a comprehensive long range mental health program. The stage is set. Despite more than a hundred years of haphazard and temporarily expedient efforts to provide custodial care for mental patients in huge isolated state mental hospitals, Missouri, like the rest of the nation, has awakened to the need, the desirability, and the wisdom of early and competent psychiatric treatment and rehabilitation at the community level.

The stage *was* set. The key actors – a compassionate governor, a sympathetic legislature, a forward-thinking and professional state mental health agency staff, and a well-educated citizenry – were in place. For the people of Missouri, the best was yet to come.

MISSOURI FIRST-PERSON INTERVIEW WITH:
HENRY "HANK" V. GUHLEMAN, M.D.

A native of Jefferson City, Dr. Hank Guhleman returned home in 1951 to begin a private practice in psychiatry and neurology. Before long he began a 30-year teaching career at the new Department of Psychiatry at the University of Missouri Medical School in Columbia, and an offer to administer the State Department of Public Health and Welfare's federal 314 (d) grant program. For more than 30 years, Hank Guhleman brought his integrity, knowledge and gentle good humor to work with him at the Department of Mental Health and its predecessor agencies.

The first board certified psychiatrist in outstate Missouri, Dr. Guhleman was a community mental health pioneer statewide. In 1985, his service to Missourians with a mental illness was recognized by the naming of the Guhleman Forensic Center at Fulton State Hospital in his honor. From 1986 to 1990, he served as a member of the Missouri Mental Health Commission

I remember going to Fulton as a kid and the patients were locked behind doors. Before reserpine all we had were the barbiturates and amphetamines. They used to mix them. Chlorpromazine was supposed to be the great drug that did everything. Of course, it had side effects.

Before that, there was insulin shock for schizophrenia and electroshock for depression. And prior to that time, they used metrazol. It was injectable; it must have been horrible. They'd inject this and pretty soon the patient would go into this terrible convulsion. My understanding was they had the erroneous idea that people with epilepsy didn't have psychiatric problems. This metrazol was refined to electroshock and insulin shock.

Insulin shock was a very elaborate treatment. The insulin shock would put them way down and then they'd give them these high doses of glucose. It was kind of hard on the veins. Sometimes the treatment took all morning. People would line up for their shock treatments all the way down the hall. There were also small doses of insulin that were sometimes used to relieve people with high anxiety.

In the beginning, the federal government didn't want to put any money into treatment for psychiatric patients until the Medicare rules came in. In 1950, the year before I arrived, they got their first 314 (d) grant here in Missouri. Each state had to have a state office designated as a mental health authority in order to receive the grant. In Missouri, the Department of Public Health and Welfare (DPHW) was designated.

Ross Gallop was the appointed head of DPHW, which was divided into divisions. Each county had a welfare board and got money for welfare. Gallop had a real "in" because all the politicians wanted money. He was quite a guy. He was very interested in mental health. The head of health, who was the man who hired me, was an Ob-gyn man with no public health experience. There were only three people in the Division of Mental Diseases[33]. The real power was with the state hospital superintendents.

In 1950, the state got its first grant and it came to the mental health authority. They didn't really know what to do with that. They made a general grant to the Health and Welfare Council of St. Louis. The story is that in St. Louis it caused so much turmoil and there was so much pressure on the council they said, "Don't do this again. You select where that money should go." And I presume that's why they [DPHW] asked me to spend one day a week with them. In 1951, we made a few grants. We used it for workshops

---

[33] The Missouri Department of Mental Health was established as a freestanding cabinet-level agency in Missouri state government in 1974. Prior to 1974, its functions were performed by the Missouri Department of Public Health and Welfare's Division of Mental Diseases (1921-1969) and Division of Mental Health (1969-1974).

with public health nurses. We did the training for discussion group leaders to work with groups who requested mental health films.

In 1952, there were no outpatient clinics of any kind associated with the state hospitals. A person was in a state hospital as a patient for years and then he left, and he was finished. The second year I was there, after we found that out, we made grants to the state hospitals so that they could start outpatient clinics. Within a few years after that, the state began to fund traveling clinics. For example, Fulton sent people up to Mexico and Mexico became a federally funded CMHC. Some of the traveling clinics got federal funding; some of them didn't. There was never a federal CMHC in Rolla, but Farmington used to send a traveling clinic to Rolla. Back when they started the community mental health centers, they had the catchment areas. That was a big deal back then. In a city like St. Louis they had a number of catchment areas of 75,000 to 200,000. My role was to go out and survey them to make sure they were in operation.

We were in a federal DHEW region, which consisted of Missouri, Iowa, Minnesota, the two Dakotas, Nebraska and Kansas. Once a year, people from the states in the region would meet in Kansas City and exchange ideas. Like I said, what we did was very primitive; we did pamphlets and workshops with people like nurses. In Iowa, they were using postmen [for casefinding], which was very interesting, especially the people who were going to where there were elderly and checking in on them.

Then all of us would go to Washington, D.C. Back in 1951, we met with people like Bob Felix at NIMH, who were housed in an office building on the mall down from the Capitol. We would share with Bob Felix what we were doing in the states. I remember the day that we had a meeting out there and they announced their community mental health concept.

When Medicare and Medicaid came along in 1965, I remember that the doctors were all upset about that; they thought that was the worst thing. The federal planners talked about it for some time before that. They weren't going to include anything for chronic

71

psychiatric patients, and the psychiatric and psychological associations got upset. A group of top-notch mental health professionals got together and said, "If we can show they're [psychiatric patients] receiving active treatment, will you reconsider?" That's when the federal people came up with the two provisions for psychiatric hospitals: they had to have adequate staffing, and their records would have to show that they had active treatment.

***MISSOURI FIRST-PERSON INTERVIEW* WITH:**

ROBIJN K. HORNSTRA, M.D.

Dr. Robijn Hornstra was born in the Netherlands and started his residency training in psychiatry at the Psychiatric Receiving Center/Kansas City General Hospitals/Greater Kansas City Mental Health Foundation in 1955. In 1958, he became a staff psychiatrist at the Foundation. In 1964, while he was the director of Adult Services at the Psychiatric Receiving Center, he was appointed the first superintendent of the Western Missouri Mental Health Center. In 1969, he became chairman of the Department of Psychiatry of the School of Medicine at the University of Missouri, Kansas City. Before his retirement in 2000, Dr. Hornstra held many positions at Western Missouri Mental Health Center in the areas of service, research and training.

In 1949, the Kansas City Association of Trusts and Foundations hired Homer Wadsworth as its director. He was a man with a vision to change the practice of medicine in the Kansas City area. He established the Greater Kansas City Mental Health Foundation in 1950. The Mental Health Foundation had a board with diverse community representation, including Kansas City (Missouri) administration, the city council, industry, banking, labor and professionals in medicine, psychiatry and law. The Trusts and Foundations provided private funding for the Mental Health Foundation's (Foundation) staffing and operations. Its mission was, and continues to be, to provide psychiatric services and mental health education, training and research.

In 1951, Kansas City contracted with the Foundation to administer the psychiatric services at each general hospital and to assist in the planning and creation of the PRC. The first director of the Mental Health Foundation was Milton Kirkpatrick, M.D., and the first clinical director was John O'Hearne, M.D. The next step was the hiring of discipline directors in social work, psychology, nursing and occupational therapy. It was also part of the plan that the child guidance clinic in Kansas City would join the Foundation staff on completion of the building.

The PRC would accept the psychiatric patients from both general hospitals[34] and the staff involved in the care at that time. The PRC was the first racially integrated facility of its kind. The NIMH gave a grant to study the integration process for two years. Two sociologists studied the integration process that turned out to be a non-event.

At the time of the opening, the services consisted of a male and female inpatient unit with a capacity of 36 patients each. There was a screening clinic staffed by social workers, psychiatrists and some psychiatric residents; a small psychotherapy clinic; and the staff of the child guidance clinic, who had important contracts with the Kansas City School District for evaluation and treatment of selected pupils. During the day, the screening clinic was open for walk-ins and appointments. The entry point in the evening was the emergency room of the general hospital. The inpatient services were supported by a milieu therapy program, hydrotherapy, insulin treatment and electroshock treatment. The professional staff were employees of the general hospital system. The support staff included the business office, the record room, the dietary department, environmental services and the psychiatric aides.

Beginning in 1955, the education, training and research activities of the Mental Health Foundation were developed. That year, the psychiatric residency training program was accredited, and the next year, Robert H. Barnes, M.D. was appointed as director of training. In 1957, we initiated training programs for senior medical students at the University of Missouri School of Medicine in Columbia. In 1958, we established a department of research with John Cumming as director. The next year, the training program in clinical psychology was accredited, and in 1960, we

---

[34] At that time, admission to general hospital care in Kansas City was segregated on the basis of race. General Hospital #1 admitted white patients and General Hospital #2 admitted African-American patients.

initiated a major group psychotherapy service and training program.

Dr. Barnes was appointed director of the Foundation when Dr. Kirkpatrick retired in 1958. That same year, the PRC aftercare clinic was established. An important aspect of this event is that the clinic initially operated only one day a week after 5 p.m., when the regular 8 to 5 staff had left. All the inpatient psychiatrists and psychiatric residents were available to see their patients. The regular outpatient staff did not participate because of their unfamiliarity with the new medications. We also established a day hospital in a small space of one inpatient floor, which was used for a small group of patients. Both the aftercare clinic and the day hospital were prompted by the gradual success with the antipsychotic medications, which were shortening hospitalizations and were capable of preventing hospital stays. As more service components became part of the service array, it was very important to adhere to a "no veto" principle once an assignment was made. No patient could be left dangling between services.

In 1961, the Foundation received the American Psychiatric Association's Mental Hospital Gold Achievement Award,

> ... for the development by the relatively small psychiatric facility of efficient, short term psychiatric services in an urban area, which a few years ago had less than minimal mental health resources. In choosing this program, the Achievement Award Committee reflected the modern trend toward hospital-community participation in a total psychiatric treatment program.

Two years later, the Foundation's overall program was designated as one of the eight model community mental health centers in the country and the NIMH awarded a demonstration grant for site visits and consultation to visitors engaged in developing comprehensive mental health centers. Also, the Missouri Legislature authorized funds for the construction and operation of a short-term treatment center for psychiatric patients in Kansas City. In 1964, ground was broken for the construction of Western

Missouri, and I was named the first superintendent. Directors of the professional disciplines at the Foundation were hired as consultants to the state Division of Mental Health to develop programs for the new Western Missouri, and in 1966, the new center was dedicated. The center's buildings consisted of the PRC connected with a bridge to the renovated former General Hospital #2, which had been gutted, and had been expanded for outpatient services. In 1968, Dr. Barnes resigned as director of the Foundation, and Charles B. Wilkinson, M.D. became the new director. I resigned as superintendent of Western Missouri to be the chairman of the Department of Psychiatry at the new University of Missouri, Kansas City School of Medicine.

MISSOURI FIRST-PERSON INTERVIEW WITH:

GEORGE A. ULETT, M.D., PH.D.

Dr. George A. Ulett is clinical professor of psychiatry at the Missouri Institute of Mental Health. From 1962-1972, Dr. Ulett was director of the Missouri Division of Mental Diseases. He has held professorships at Washington University and St. Louis University Schools of Medicine and was professor and chairman of the Department of Psychiatry at the Missouri Institute of Psychiatry at the University of Missouri School of Medicine. He is the author of 270 scholarly articles and books.

When I took over as director of the Division of Mental Diseases, it was with great reluctance. I said I would take the job for six months. I was director of Malcolm Bliss and a professor at Washington University. I had a tenured position and I was just having a ball. We were doing a lot of research and were turning out dozens of papers. I went down to Bliss to see what electroshock was all about. In those days, curare was just coming in. At Malcolm Bliss, everybody got electroconvulsive therapy. They had four husky guys hold the patients down to do it. Dr. Kathleen Smith and I went down there to see what was going on.

I was sitting with my feet up on the desk eating a sandwich one day when a fellow came in with a bow tie and a dark suit on and said, "I'm John Dalton." I nearly fell out of the chair. I knew he was the governor but I had never seen him. He asked me a few questions about mental health. He said he had heard about our new program at Bliss and I said we had brought residents down from Wash. U., and that it had been neglected since it was built with WPA funds in 1937. The patients were all getting shock therapy and nobody was getting proper treatment. The nurses were using this as a training center on how to put people in wet sheet packs and how to do hydrotherapy. We brought resident psychiatrists as doctors to treat people and the new drugs were coming in. So he said, "I just wanted to meet you."

Well, seven or eight months later all hell broke loose and Dr. Addison Duval was gone. The governor was looking for someone to replace him and asked me to have lunch with him. Since he'd been asking me questions about mental health, I thought he called me out there to help him find somebody. Just as we finished lunch, he said, "By the way, I'd really like you to take this job." We walked out of the room and met with all the reporters and he said, "I just asked Dr. Ulett to take this job." And they asked if I was going to take it, and I said I'd have to think about it.

I knew I could get a sabbatical from Wash. U. for six months, but if I took the state job full time, I would have to give up my tenured professorship there. I decided I was not going to take it. The next day I got a call from Al Baur who was the superintendent at Fulton and he said, "George, I know you've been asked to take the job and I know you're thinking of turning it down, but before you say, "No," would you come out and visit me?"

I drove to Fulton and Al Baur took me down to the basement of one of the buildings and said,

> You see this ward? When I came here, there were 35 patients sitting in these steel rocking chairs. From each chair there was chiseled a channel going down to the central drain. The patients were brought in here and they were shackled into the chairs at seven in the morning and they were not unshackled until eight at night. They ate in the chairs, and they were not even released to empty their bowels or bladders. The attendant, who was a farm worker, came through with a hose the way they did at the farm and hosed the place out every few hours. If you don't take that job, these conditions will revert, and it will be just like that again. All the good people Duval brought in will leave. No one will come to Missouri after the firing of the director by the governor. It will look bad. Will you take it temporarily?

I said, "Well I could take it for six months while they find somebody." He said, "Okay, do that." I said I would take it temporarily, but only for six months.

All of a sudden I found out what I was into: 10,000 patients, and only a handful of doctors. I said what this place really needs is what I did at Malcolm Bliss; we need to get doctors in here. So I sat down with Mont Hardwicke and Hank Guhleman, because they knew the state and I didn't, and I said, "What do I do?" And they asked, "What do you want to do?" I said, "Well, the best thing I can do is start training doctors. You can't hire doctors to work in the state hospitals; they don't want to get involved with chronic patients. If I could set up my own residency training program and offer doctors more money than the other residency programs in the state can, I'll make it a career program so that they're indebted to me for two years of service and we won't give them all of their five years of training credit until they're through. With this, I can get doctors from all over the world to come here." So they said, "What do you need to do this? I said, "Well, I need some money and I need a building." They said, "Go to the governor. He's in your debt. He wants to hold you up and say, 'See what I got. He's a good guy and he can turn this thing around'."

I told the governor, "I want to build a school for doctors to work in these hospitals." He asked what I needed, and I told him that I needed a new building and about a half-million dollars. He said, "There's a new building there in St. Louis that was built as an overflow for TB patients and they really don't need it for that use. I'll just tell them to give you that building and I have a half-million dollars in my contingency fund, so go ahead and start your school." We got it off the ground, and the Missouri Institute of Psychiatry[35] (MIP) was our major center for residency training and research on new drugs. In ten years, we trained 125 doctors and we sent them around to the hospitals. We also published over 100 research papers at MIP.

---

[35] Now known as the Missouri Institute of Mental Health.

The faculty added greatly to our overall program. An example was the Gheel [Belgium] type community program suggested to me and organized by Dr. Ali Keskiner. We selected the small river town of New Haven as our experimental community. Two local clergy got the local government to approve the town becoming a "mental hospital without walls." We were the first in the U.S. to try this. We introduced patients to the townsfolk with ice cream socials and other events. Ultimately, 25 patients came to live with 25 families. When I surveyed the town 20 years later, I found that none of the patients had ever gone back into the hospital. Some had gone home; others with physical ailments entered nursing homes; a few were still living in the town. Had I stayed with the program longer, I planned to develop Gheel-type programs in other small Missouri towns. I lost my tenure at Wash. U., but I did not care as I was so excited about what I was doing. I stepped into a helluva problem.

I wanted to bring in more residents and I went up to the osteopathic college in Kirksville and met with the chairman of psychiatry and I said, "What do you do for the training of your psychiatrists?" She said, "We have to send them to France." I said, "How would you like to have a residency program here in the United States? I'll turn over one of my state hospitals to you." I called Dr. Paul Barone down at Nevada and he was excited about having residents come down there. I said I would have them rotate for part of the time through MIP, and she said that was great. I had to run this past the state medical society. At their next council meeting I said I wanted to start training osteopaths. This was 1969, and they still hadn't settled the problem of D.O.s at that time. They said I couldn't do that. I said, "Look, I have 10,000 patients and a dozen doctors; if you'll give me a dozen doctors for my state hospitals, I'll forget about the osteopaths." They said, "No, we can't do that." I said, "Okay then, I have to have them." They debated and I brought the osteopaths in. We broke that bottleneck.

I stayed on with Governor Dalton who had only two years to go. Then Governor Hearnes came in. Warren Hearnes had been active in the MHA; he was very much a mental health governor. On my

Mental Health Commission, I had Jack Stapleton, a newspaper owner from Dunklin County who was very close to the governor. We were all set to go. Our budget was always favored over other budgets. I had a wonderful [state mental health] commission. I also had Dr. Margaret Gildea, a Jungian trained psychiatrist and wife of the psychiatry department chairman at Wash. U., and Dr. Bob Felix, who had been chief of NIMH in Washington, D.C.

The finest thing I ever did in my entire career was to break the segregation – black and white – in the City of St. Louis. I was the head of Malcolm Bliss for about three years. Mayor Tucker decided to make me the head of psychiatry for the City of St. Louis. They had a psychiatric unit at Homer Phillips, the black hospital. I went over there and I was shocked. They had one hall for their psychiatry unit. At night they brought folding beds up out of the basement and the patients slept head to toe because it was so overcrowded. I said we had empty space at Malcolm Bliss; we could make new wards there. So I went to the mayor and said I wanted to consolidate these programs. He said, "We're having a big battle now; they're trying to close Homer Phillips and if you take one service out of that hospital, why that will be the collapse of it." So I went to the hospital commissioner and said I could not be the head of psychiatry in St. Louis with a segregated service. "We've got to do something about this." I told him what the mayor said. "Well," he said, "I'll tell you what we're going to do. I'll phone the ambulance headquarters and tell them that all acute psychiatric cases, regardless of their skin color, come to Malcolm Bliss." So then it was black and white on mixed wards, and this soon brought integration to St. Louis State Hospital.

When I came to the division, I wanted to do a Malcolm Bliss type program in three parts of the state. I went over to Kansas City and met with Dr. Robijn Hornstra and saw what they were doing over there and I became excited because we already had acute admission treatment and training possibilities at two ends of the state, and then I came in for Columbia in the middle. We were ready to dig the ground for a similar unit in Columbia at Mid-MO when the federal money came through. Western Missouri was operational with private funding. When I sold the legislators on the three centers, I had a picture with lines going out from each to rural communities. My idea was to have traveling clinics go out to these rural communities. This helped sell the concept with the rural legislators, with all these spokes going out to their hometowns. I was not around long enough to get that program going. I was busy training doctors, and I knew that they would get around to that naturally.

The new drugs were coming. The medications were really the key to being able to return patients to the community. I know up to that time there was no control of their symptoms. The drugs were there and I needed the doctors to administer the drugs. As new drugs to treat mental illness were becoming available, I needed to stress a psychiatric treatment program. I recruited a psychiatrist to head each of the seven major hospitals and three acute treatment centers.

We had a good administrative staff that made the program successful. Melded into a team with each of these physicians was a good business manager to jointly run the hospital. All these teams met with me each month at the various hospitals. As a governing body, they made plans and assisted me in handling the problems at the various institutions. I met with the mental health commission each month, also at a different hospital, and brought them up to date on our planning. In addition, in the central office I had a chief business manager, Dave Roberts; a chief social worker, Ed Davis; a chief of psychology and outpatient clinics, Dick Cravens; and other heads of nursing and dietary.

With the assistance of these fine professionals, the program shifted its focus from custodial to treatment. During my tenure, we dropped the chronic hospital population from 10,000 patients to 5,000. We built two hospitals for children with mental illness and started small units around the state for persons with mental retardation and other disabilities. With the help of Dr. Joseph Kendis in St. Louis, we started treatment units for alcohol and drug addiction. I stayed on a total of ten years before leaving for private practice.

WARREN HEARNES: In the early 1950s, I became acquainted with some people who were interested in mental health. We had what I called the civilian board, who weren't paid for by anyone: David Skeer, Jack Stapleton, Helen Twersky. We met in St. Louis, Kansas City and different places and became sort of rabid with interest in mental health. That was the lead as far as my interest in mental health in the early 1950s.

I started in the legislature in 1951 at the ripe old age of 27. The traveling clinics were an issue in 1955. By the time 1955 came along, I thought I was a seasoned veteran. I did have four years in and knew my way around by that time. It made it a lot easier, you know, because the more longevity you have in the legislature, the better you can serve. I always heard there was so much animosity between the rural and the urban areas, and I preached all the time that it's all one state. I always used for an example in St. Louis, "Where do you think all these people that go to the Cardinals baseball games come from?" They come from rural areas in Missouri and Illinois. I could get through to them that way.

If you could take the whole state, the mental health situation was not good at all. In every mental health department in every state, you always had the same problem: money. And you can say all you want about this, if you do not have the money, you can't take care of the patients. That's something the average person (unless they're interested in mental health, as I was), who doesn't have a tie to mental health with a family member in need, does not fully understand. The legislators are like these average people. Unless they're on a certain committee, they do not have that knowledge. They don't understand that when you cut mental health, you're cutting patients.

The traveling clinics were about the only help the rural people had; they were precursors of the later community-based services. Before the traveling clinics and the intensive treatment centers and regional diagnostic centers, parents had no place to go for diagnosis and treatment.

BETTY HEARNES: In his first message to the Missouri General Assembly in 1965, Warren recommended maximum financial support for the three intensive treatment centers in St. Louis, Columbia and Kansas City authorized by the 72nd General Assembly. His first recommendation was the establishment and support of nine regional diagnostic and treatment clinics for the mentally retarded. And of course, that was just the start of those with the nine; two more followed. I'm putting words in his mouth, but it was very important for the intensive treatment centers to be fully financed; we were still with the traveling clinics, and that's why Warren was trying to do the nine diagnostic centers. To

Warren, that meant that everybody would be within an hour of treatment, and that's what he told the General Assembly.

Jack (Stapleton) and George (Ulett) had the plan. Jack had worked with Warren and David Skeer and Helen Twersky and several doctors and they had been on what Warren called the civilian board, with no authority at all and no pay, and that was a forerunner of the Mental Health Commission. I believed that Jack and George had worked on this plan themselves to get what Warren wanted. Warren wanted to give treatment to the whole state. Of course, he had worked on that in the General Assembly. Warren was impressed with the plan because it was going to meet some needs for people all over the state of Missouri that they never had met before, even with the traveling clinics.

WARREN HEARNES: As far as the legislature is concerned, when you lead off a message with something, they know it has a lot behind it. It gets much more attention when it comes off first than when it comes halfway through the speech. There was talk in political circles about the state of mental health in Missouri, and there were those who said that it was the second worst in the United States. Now that's easy to say, that kind of talk. But when you see everything that's been done, whether it was in my administration or other administrations or what, it had to be in bad shape when I was elected governor.

BETTY HEARNES: In 1951, I recall that if you had a child that you couldn't handle and you couldn't do anything with, and the child had a psychiatric problem, you had one thing you could do. You could lock him upstairs in his bedroom, and that was it. As far as I can remember, there wasn't any place to go. And I think that's what Warren saw, and what that civilian board saw, that things were in terrible shape in mental health in Missouri.

Everything has changed since Warren was in the governor's office. I think some of the community mental health centers are doing great. For example, Myra Callahan is doing a terrific job. At one time I was on the board of Ron Steinmetz's center, Bootheel Counseling Services. But I am still concerned that with the people with a mental illness in the community, we must have the staff to make sure that they're taking their medicine and so forth.

One of the things I worked on while I was on the Mental Health Commission was accessibility, because I come from a rural area. Let me say this, the way we give the service has changed tremendously. Up until all of these cuts, I think we were doing very well. I don't know what is going to happen now. We'll just have to wait and see what level of service they can give.

Child mental health concerns have exploded. In California, they report a 200% increase in autistic children, and some slough it off saying, "Now we can diagnose this better." I don't think that's right. I taught school in the 1950s and in the 1960s, and I did not see a child in my room that manifested those characteristics that I see in an autistic child. I know what I'm looking for when I see an autistic child, and that is what concerns me most of all because it has just exploded. In this small town, where we would never see a child with autism before, we do see them now. I'm not talking about children with learning difficulties. With the parent advisory groups throughout the state, with the money that comes for that, we are making some progress here in Missouri. I chair the parent group in southeast Missouri, even though I am not a parent, and we serve 250 families in 19 counties. That's a lot of kids. I'm looking for a cure.

4 THE GROWTH OF PRIVATE COMMUNITY MENTAL HEALTH CENTERS (1967-1980)

The seeds of private CMHCs in Missouri were planted in 1955, when the Missouri General Assembly required that state hospitals dispatch traveling clinics to local, especially rural, communities. Nurtured by Division of Mental Diseases staff experienced in writing grants for federal CMHC funding, these seeds bore fruit beginning in 1967 with the opening of the federally funded East Central Missouri Mental Health Center[36] in Mexico, Missouri. By the end of 1981, federally funded CMHCs sponsored by private, not-for-profit agencies were added in communities surrounding Joplin, Cape Girardeau, Hannibal, Springfield, St. Joseph and St. Charles, as well as four new CMHCs in the greater Kansas City area and one in St. Louis. At the same time, other outreach clinics, now fully under local control, began to reach out, expanding their service offerings.

Arthur Center

In their *Missouri First-Person Interviews*, Dick Cravens [pp. 119-124] and East Central's first executive director, Jack Viar [pp. 125-131], recall he origins of this groundbreaking center. A traveling

---

[36] As dynamic organizations, from time to time Missouri CMHCs change their corporate names to best reflect the roles that they play in their changing communities. For example, East Central is now known as Arthur Center.

clinic from Fulton State Hospital formed the nucleus of clinical care and administrative expertise in this community, around which local leaders pushed for the development of a comprehensive CMHC. A sympathetic administrator at the local Audrain County Hospital, with the backing of his board of directors, attempted to garner federal CMHC construction funds. Unsuccessful at first, he enlisted the traveling clinic's social worker to prepare a successful application in his free time.

Over the past 35 years, the operation has grown to include a full range of mental health services from outpatient to case management to inpatient care. It operates both supported living and supported employment programs for persons who need rehabilitation services to support their re-entry into community life. Renamed in 1997 to honor J. B. Arthur, a local business leader and philanthropist, it has been designated by DMH as the administrative agent[37] for the service area comprised of Audrain, Callaway, Monroe, Montgomery, Pike and Ralls counties. In 2003, Chief Executive Officer (CEO) Terry Mackey, center employees and interested citizens orchestrated the decoupling of Arthur Center from Audrain Medical Center, while continuing to provide a comprehensive mental health program in its six-county area.

Ozark Center

At about the same time, mental health professionals and private citizens in far southwest Missouri were planning a federally funded CMHC of their own. In 1961, the Western Jasper County MHA organized an outpatient mental health clinic in Joplin, a forerunner both of the CMHC currently headquartered in that city and of centers nationwide. It opened in 1962 in a frame building provided by Freeman Hospital, which accepted legal responsibility for all of the clinic's debts [43]. In 1965, the clinic was transferred to the

---

[37] In 1981, DMH designated one mental health entity within each service area to receive the department's purchase of service (POS) funding for all mental illness services provided in its designated area and to serve as the entry-exit point for admission to and discharge from state mental hospitals.

Ozark Psychiatric Foundation. In the same year, representatives of the Eastern Jasper County MHA successfully negotiated with the Missouri Division of Mental Diseases to dispatch a traveling clinic from Nevada State Hospital. This aftercare clinic for former state hospital patients was located in a house provided by the MHA adjacent to McCune-Brooks Hospital in Carthage. From this broad base of experience and community awareness, citizens in Barton, Jasper, Newton and McDonald counties formed a new board of directors and submitted applications for both federal CMHC construction and staffing grants in 1969. Both grants were approved, and the Ozark Community Mental Health Center (OCMHC) opened in 1969 on land donated by St. John's Regional Medical Center, which also provided the needed inpatient services under contract. That building remains in use today. Over the next seven years, clinics were opened in Neosho, Pineville and Lamar, and emergency services were organized through a volunteer hotline. When the center's staffing grant drew to a close in 1977, it had a staff of eight, a $300,000 budget, one building, 300 patients, and a new CEO: Michael B. Cole, Ph.D.

Cole and his staff led the way for many of the Missouri CMHCs. In 1978, OCMHC obtained the first DMH purchase-of-service (POS) contract for mental health services. This contract helped OCMHC maintain its budget and level of care, while allowing room for growth. In the same year, the Missouri Coalition of Community Mental Health Centers,[38] then chaired by Cole, successfully lobbied the state legislature to liberalize property tax statutes for mental health services, allowing a simple majority vote in any county or political subdivision for a tax to be levied. Newton and Jasper counties passed the first two property taxes for mental health services in Missouri, the benefits of which continue to date, locally and statewide. Funding for substance abuse services formerly offered at Nevada State Hospital was awarded to

---

[38] The Missouri Coalition of Community Mental Health Centers was started as an informal association of the state's private CMHCs in the early 1970s. Incorporated on July 10, 1978, its first employee was Kathy Carter, once a member of the OCMHC board of directors. Ms. Carter was hired in September 1979, and has been the Coalition's CEO through the present.

OCMHC, which opened a substance abuse program called *New Directions*, offering detoxification, residential treatment, and outpatient counseling.

More than 25 years later, OCMHC, since renamed Ozark Center, has added services including: a psychosocial rehabilitation program and independent living services for adults with serious and persistent mental illness who had received service at Nevada State hospital; a comprehensive psychiatric treatment facility for children with an emotional disturbance; a residential care facility with a psychiatric care component; and a pharmacy whose exclusive purpose is dispensing psychiatric medications to patients.

In 1996, Ozark Center became an affiliate of the 3,400 employee Freeman Health System. As the exclusive behavioral health provider for Freeman Health System, Ozark Center has developed and manages an acute adult psychiatric unit and a geriatric psychiatric unit, while managing nine psychiatric practices with distinctive competencies in child and adolescent psychiatry, geriatric psychiatry, adult psychiatry, and hospital consultation/ liaison services. Ozark Center has enjoyed 10% growth per year in patients and revenue since deploying its system of behavioral healthcare integrated with primary care. It provides services to over 10,000 patients annually. Ozark Center still serves as DMH's agent in Barton, Jasper, Newton, and McDonald counties. The center now employs 350 staff; owns, operates or manages 160 beds; occupies 18 facilities; and has an annual budget of $25 million and a seasoned CEO: Dr. Mike Cole.

Tri-County Mental Health Services

The location of its mental hospitals in rural Missouri at first worked a hardship on persons with a mental illness residing in the more populated areas of St. Louis and Jackson counties. St. Louis solved the accessibility problem by building a municipal mental health facility in 1869. Until the mid 1950s, the citizens of Kansas City and surrounding Jackson County relied primarily on St. Joseph State Hospital, up to 75 miles away, for intensive mental health care. While an early liability, the lack of a local mental hospital provided a clear field for the development of private CMHCs in the greater Kansas City area. The first of these was Tri-County Mental Health Center, opened in North Kansas City in 1973. In their *Missouri First-Person Interviews*, Jack Viar [pp. 125-131] Tri-County's first executive director, and Morty Lebedun [pp. 133-141], current CEO, recount the early days at Tri-County.

Prior to 1973, this area north of the Missouri River was served by an outreach clinic from Western MO. In 1971, Tony McCanna, social service director at North Kansas City Hospital, prepared federal CMHC staffing and construction grant applications, which were submitted by the hospital. Both were awarded in 1972, and construction was begun shortly thereafter. Tri-County's new building was a source of community pride in the Clay, Platte and Ray county area. The center started as a hospital-based service that included a 24-bed inpatient unit. Over 100 staff members were hired to operate programs at the main facility and at satellite clinics established in rural areas like Richmond and Platte City. The center also established a 19-bed drug rehabilitation unit in 1974 and became known as a quality service provider with a full array of mandated services including prevention and education. The termination of Tri-County's federal staffing grant coincided with DMH's increased focus on local services for persons with serious and persistent mental illnesses. In 1989, the hospital withdrew[39] from its role as the primary provider of publicly supported mental health services in its service area.

---

[39] According to Charles Ray [87], North Kansas City Hospital was required to buy out of the mental health service obligation it accepted for receiving federal construction funds. Their remaining balance due was $1,050,000. In 1991, they paid $800,000, with Tri-County and the levy board making up the rest. According to Lebedun [67], "That million dollars was put in escrow to create our new building. We raised another million and constructed the Northland Human Services Building on the campus of Maple Woods. We moved in June 1995, and Charles Ray was the dedication speaker at the event." Ray, a former employee of North Kansas City Hospital, was president and CEO of the National Council for Community Behavioral Healthcare, a position he continues to hold. North Kansas City Hospital remains an important community partner of Tri-County to the present time.

In 1990, interested citizens regrouped and formed a new corporation, Tri-County Mental Health Services, Inc. Since then, this agency has grown to serve 8,000 consumers each year with a budget of $8 million and a staff of 67. Recently developed services include 18 housing units, drug courts, prevention programs in 15 school districts and mobile crisis interventions at local hospitals and consumers' homes. A skill center is being built to expand vocational services and day programs and to provide a home for the consumer-run drop-in center.

Based on a brokered services approach first developed in 1983 by DMH's Great Rivers Mental Health Services in St. Louis County and a private managed mental health agency in Kansas City, the new Tri-County aggressively recruited private mental health professionals to serve area residents under its auspices. Although the balance of purchased to provided services has shifted from 80%-20% in 1990 to near 50%-50% today, the agency contracts with at least 75 providers and service organizations in a networked system that treats clients in their home community. The Tri-County network approach is recognized as a prototype for cost-effective CMHCs of the future.

ReDiscover (formerly Research Mental Health Services)

First known as the Southeastern Jackson County Community Mental Health Center, this agency was started in 1968 in classrooms at Unity Village with a 314 (d) grant from DMH. Staffed by volunteers, with professional staff from Western MO and Family and Children's Services, it was also given space for 14 inpatient beds at the old Jackson County Public Hospital (now Truman Medical Center-Lakewood). In 1972, a federal CMHC construction grant was awarded, and the new center's opening in 1974 coincided with the arrival of federal staffing funds.

Led from 1973 to 1994 by Shirley Fearon, a community-oriented nurse, the center exemplifies the flexibility of the CMHC approach. In addition to providing the services required under the federal funding requirements, the center developed and ran client businesses, responded to disasters in its home community and around the country, and designed *What's the Secret?*, a child sexual abuse prevention program that is utilized in 68 schools. Personal accounts of the history of the center are provided in the *Missouri First-Person Interviews* with Shirley Fearon [pp.143-148] and longtime board member, Doug Hall [pp. 149-152].

In 1977, the center's name was shortened to Community Mental Health Center-South. In 1984, it merged with Research Health Services, a partnership that extended for 19 years, until the recent sale of the parent health system (Health Midwest) to Hospital Corporation of America. Freestanding once again, the center continues its work with vitality and vision. Now known as ReDiscover, but still under the leadership of CEO Alan Flory, the center has an annual budget of $12 million. Its 260 employees provide services to 7,000 consumers annually at five sites and in home-based, school-based, jail-based and office-based settings. Services include a full range of outpatient, residential, 24-hour crisis, and partial hospital care, as well as prevention services for addictions and mental health.

Comprehensive Mental Health Services

Thirty-five years ago, the director of the Independence health department approached administrators from Independence Sanitarium and Hospital about the mental health needs of the community. In 1969, the Independence Area Mental Health Center was incorporated and leased space for a small outpatient clinic from the hospital. Staff from Western MO provided outpatient care for adults and children and day activities for adults, and the Junior Service League of Independence funded a therapist for children's mental health needs.

In 1972, the agency's name was changed to Northeastern Jackson County Mental Health Center to more appropriately reflect the geographic area it served, and a small 314 (d) grant was awarded by the Division of Mental Diseases. The next year, patient fees and grants from community organizations and Jackson County allowed the hiring of the first permanent staff members: a part-time psychiatric nurse who worked with children, executive director John Macek, and a part-time medical director. Federal CMHC staffing grant funding became available in mid-1974. Staff members were hired to provide the required five services: inpatient, outpatient, partial hospital, emergency services, and consultation and education. The following year, an outpatient office opened in Blue Springs, the first of many new center sites.

The years between 1978 and 1983 were a watershed for this burgeoning mental health agency. In July 1978, the board hired Dr. James McKee as executive director. Three months later, William H. Kyles joined as associate director. Picked to replace McKee in 1982, Kyles has shared his observations on mental health services in Jackson County and Missouri in his *Missouri First-Person Interview* [pp. 153-160]. Certification to provide alcohol and drug abuse services, DMH POS and community placement contracts, and the passage of the first Jackson County Mental Health Levy protected the newly named Comprehensive Mental Health Services, Inc. (CMHS) from the impact of declining federal financial support and projected it in new directions.

In the intervening 20 years, CMHS has made great advances under the leadership of its board and CEO Bill Kyles. Two of these are worthy of special notice. From 1983 to 1993, CMHS was a prime participant in the federal government's Cuban Refugee Resettlement Program, offering treatment, housing, and vocational training to Cubans with mental illness. This was one of very few federal grants awarded for mental health services for refugees of the *Mariel Boatlift*, and the only one in Missouri. Second, in 1998, Renaissance West, a highly visible and important 30-year-old inner-city substance abuse program, was acquired by CMHS as a subsidiary corporation.

This center continues to serve the people of northeastern Jackson County as well as the inner city of Kansas City, Missouri. Approximately 200 staff serve about 4,000 clients per year. Started with $1,700 in local contributions, 35 years later it has an annual budget of $10 million.

Swope Health Services

All of Jackson County's catchment areas became recipients of federal CMHC grants with the establishment of the CMHC at the Model Cities Comprehensive Neighborhood Health Center on Linwood Boulevard in Kansas City, Missouri. This federally qualified health center began in 1970 in a church basement with a modest $65,000 grant and the leadership of E. Frank Ellis. The fledgling organization expanded over the years into Swope Health Enterprises, which includes an HMO, a community development corporation, a federally qualified health center, a CMHC, and an urban planning and research arm.

The CMHC opened in 1980 on Swope Parkway. Its first program director, Brenda Pelofsky, was responsible for developing and implementing the initial array of mental health services with a staff of five employees. These early services included partial/day treatment services, and community living skills. Later, case management services were added. Drs. Curtis Franklin and Dasari Ratnam were instrumental in developing the early psychiatric services.

Swope faced immediate obstacles in providing mental health services to the predominantly African-American population they served. The stigma of seeking mental health treatment – in addition to poverty and minority status – prevented many from seeking needed care. To address these barriers, Swope carried the message of community mental health to churches, schools and other natural helping institutions where African Americans traditionally sought help. Programs were designed, named and marketed with the target population in mind. Swope became a training ground for African-American mental health professionals. These efforts aligned well with the center's mission to improve the physical, mental, economic and spiritual health of the community.

Dianne Cleaver, who had served as a center supervisor, became the director in 1985. Shortly thereafter, the agency was renamed the Swope Parkway Health Center. During Cleaver's tenure, programs were expanded and new programs were launched. She was involved in the passage of the Jackson County Mental Health Levy

Fund and was a founder of CommCare, the Community Network for Behavioral Healthcare.

In 1991, efforts to establish a drug rehabilitation center met with resistance from the surrounding neighborhoods of Sheraton Estates and Mount Cleveland. Swope pledged to clear the neighborhood of drug houses and crime, and residents endorsed the building of Imani[40] House, Swope's 30-bed residential treatment center for adults. One of the few culturally specific programs in Missouri, and state funded, Imani House was designed to address the recovery needs of African-Americans and individuals who were impacted by HIV/AIDs. Funds from Jackson County's one-quarter cent sales tax were used to shore up the funding needed to operate and sustain the program. Also in 1991, stable, supportive housing was established for persons with serious and persistent mental illness who had been residing at St. Joseph State Hospital.

In 1995, a $21.3 million development project was completed and community mental health services were relocated into state-of-the-art facilities in two buildings of the new complex. In 1997, clinical psychologist Susan B. Wilson, Ph.D. was named director of the behavioral health division. Under her leadership, services and revenues were expanded once more to include adolescent drug treatment, a children's psychiatric rehabilitation program, mental health court services, faith-based and school-based substance abuse prevention programs, and services for senior adults. Swope Parkway's mental health center currently operates with a budget of $8.9 million and a staff of 150.

Hopewell Center

Across the state in St. Louis, a similar enterprise was unfolding at the same time. Hopewell Center traces its roots to north St. Louis City residents who wished to serve the health care needs of the poor, elderly and disabled persons in their medically and economically underserved communities. In 1969, federal funds were

---

[40] The name "Imani' is a Kiswahili word meaning "faith."

awarded to the Yeatman District Community Corporation, establishing the Yeatman Health Center, a comprehensive health center, on North Grand Boulevard in St. Louis. Later, the Yeatman/Union-Sarah Joint Commission on Health Care, Inc. was formed, and the Union-Sarah Center, on Delmar Boulevard, opened its doors in 1972. This center provided health services in a dramatically underserved area, and was an engine for promoting economic growth and opportunities for the community it served. It offered many social support services, childcare, transportation, job training and housing assistance.

In 1979, the corporation was awarded a $700,000 comprehensive mental health services grant. Dr. Amanda L. Murphy was selected to head the new mental health center, and she has served as its president and chief executive officer since 1980. A measure of the mental health center's relevance to its community was apparent in the observations of Norman J. Tice [103], then president of nearby City Bank, and chairman of the Missouri Mental Health Commission:

> As far as I was concerned, they were getting services to persons in low-income areas that had no services. It was one of the forerunners. In those days you had to go to the people, and this center did just that.

In 1985, the agency's name was changed to Metro Comprehensive Mental Health Center. Three years later, the parent corporation transferred the mental health center's assets to Hopewell Center.

The center's philosophy and values are consistent with the Balanced Services System Model. A multidisciplinary staff of 130 provide a rich panel of 28 well-integrated, culturally competent services of high quality to 4,500 patients yearly. Approximately 89% of its clients classify themselves as African-American.

Over the years, Hopewell has moved its services outside the clinic walls. Today, more than 50% of the center's services are provided in natural environments such as schools, homes and other residential settings. A large percentage of Hopewell Center's $7.5

million annual budget is set aside to serve persons with a mental illness who are unable to pay for their own treatment. Other funding sources include the federal government, foundations and other private sources, local tax dollars, insurance and patient fees. Ongoing attention is given to maximizing resources and participating in development efforts to raise funds, thereby decreasing dependency on state and federal funds.

In May 2003, Murphy was recognized for her lifelong dedication to providing high-quality services to the residents of her community. At that time, she was interviewed in her Hopewell office by Tavia Evans of the *St. Louis American* newspaper [28]. Surrounded by souvenirs of her journeys to other lands where life routinely challenges people, she gave a 2003 voice to the reason that dedicated mental health professionals have chosen to serve others in their communities for more than 240 years:

> 'We try to give people back the dignity they need, to keep them feeling strong enough to...put their lives back together.' She paused, glancing at the photos from faraway places. 'We don't get into these professions by accident; we really want to help people.'

Community Counseling Center

For nearly 30 years, the citizens of Bollinger, Cape Girardeau, Madison, Perry and Ste. Genevieve counties in Missouri have been the beneficiaries of the vision of three determined women. Sister Virgilia Beikler, OSF, administrator of Cape Girardeau's St. Francis Hospital during the 1970s, was concerned that the hospital did not offer much assistance to children with an emotional disturbance or to adults with a mental illness.

At the same time, Jeannette Boehme, a counselor at Perryville High School, worked with disturbed teenagers who came from dysfunctional homes. She wished for a mental health clinic to which she could refer children and families who needed more help than school counselors could provide. Boehme and Evelyn Hinni, a local parochial school teacher, made a phone call to inquire about mental health programs at Saint Francis Hospital. It was a call that Sister Virgilia would answer in more ways than one. The three women met and soon realized that they all shared the same dream of providing community counseling for the mentally ill. Sister Virgilia hired Lou Masterman, a longtime consultant on community mental health programs, to write a grant application requesting federal CMHC funds for the hospital and surrounding five counties. Their efforts were successful, and St. Francis Mental Health Center began its important work in 1974, with Masterman as its first director.

The center began amid modest accommodations – a picnic table and two chairs – in the little brick house where the nuns used to live at the old Saint Francis Hospital grounds on South Ellis Street. Volunteer counselors began meeting with clients, and a 24-hour crisis hotline was set up. This preliminary work set a solid foundation for the center's future growth. Construction on the new facility began in 1973, and concerns about receiving federal operating funds prompted the board of directors to open the center early, in the old hospital facility, to assure their receipt. Initially, 34 staff members were hired. Once the new facility was completed in fall 1976, the center's new director, Dr. Morty Lebedun, hired 20 more. Lebedun recalls his experiences in Cape Girardeau in his *Missouri First-Person Interview* [pp. 133-141].

In January 1985, the center became the independent entity now known as Community Counseling Center. Presently, center CEO John Hudak oversees the staff of 170, who serve 5,000 patients annually in eight facilities, with full-time clinics in each of its five counties. They maintain a continuum of 14 services, including psychiatry, outpatient, community-based services for adults and children, intensive in-home services, psychosocial rehabilitation, a consumer managed and staffed warm line, and a transitional living group home for adults and crisis services. It has an annual budget in excess of $6.5 million.

Mark Twain Area Counseling Center

The mid-1970s was a period of growth for private federally funded CMHCs in all regions of Missouri. In 1975, the Mark Twain Mental Health Center opened in Hannibal, Missouri, the town Samuel Clemens made famous. An outgrowth of the organizing efforts of the Mark Twain Association for Mental Health, Inc., the new center built on the earlier services provided by a traveling clinic dispatched from Fulton State Hospital. A satellite office was opened in Kirksville shortly thereafter and was called Kirksville Counseling Clinic. Over the years, clinics were also opened in Macon and Memphis, Missouri. When federal funds were reduced in 1981, Mark Twain successfully pursued POS funding through DMH. At that time Mark Twain became the administrative agent for the nine northeast counties of Missouri: Adair, Clark, Knox, Lewis, Macon, Marion, Schuyler, Scotland and Shelby. By 1990, the center had closed all satellite offices except Kirksville, serving all the surrounding counties via traveling clinics based out of the two full-time offices. The center's name was changed at that time to the Mark Twain Area Counseling Center (MTACC).

Currently, the 70 MTACC staff serve more than 2,000 consumers annually throughout its nine-county service area. With a $3.2 million annual budget, the center offers an array of affordable behavioral health services to the citizens of northeast Missouri, including outpatient services for children, adults, and families experiencing difficulties with life issues. Specialized services are available through MTACC's community psychiatric rehabilitation (CPR) program for adults and children experiencing a severe disabling mental illness. Children's services are offered in the home, school and office. Intensive in-home services are available to families coping with a child with a serious emotional disturbance. MTACC offers a 24-hour crisis intervention system with a mobile response capability. Crisis intervention staff respond to local law enforcement and to hospital emergency departments as well as to private individuals and families. Psychiatric evaluations, medication services, psychotherapy, consultation, and a variety of educational programs for community agencies are routinely available. Under the leadership of Executive Director Pat Murdock,

MTACC continues to participate in multiple interagency councils, partnerships and collaborative efforts in helping serve the mental health needs in the region.

Burrell Behavioral Health

Like its counterpart in Joplin, Burrell Behavioral Health in Springfield has a long and distinguished history of service to an area of Missouri that previously lacked comprehensive and accessible mental health services. Cravens [pp. 119-124], in his *Missouri First-Person Interview*, recounts the early history of Burrell, which is told in greater detail by Dr. Todd Schaible [pp. 161-168], the center's only CEO, in his *Interview*. A federal CMHC staffing grant was approved in 1976, and Burrell's first client was seen in May 1977 in the center's main office in the Empire Building on South Avenue in Springfield. Other offices soon followed in Buffalo, Bolivar, Greenfield and Marshfield. Inpatient services were provided under an agreement with Park Central Hospital. Other services included outpatient, substance abuse, adult treatment and 24-hour emergency.

The following year, the service array was expanded to include children's day treatment, consultation and education, and case management for nursing and boarding homes. The center's first POS contract with DMH, specialized services for persons with a serious mental illness, an independent living apartment program and employee assistance services followed in 1979. Soon, residential services were added and case management services expanded; a merger with Lakes Area Counseling Services extended services to Christian, Stone and Taney counties.

In the early 1980s, frustrated in its efforts to find a permanent home, Burrell entered into a remarkable series of real estate transactions in an undeveloped section of south Springfield. In 1985, Burrell moved into a new state-of-the-art facility overlooking Burrell Park in the heart of what is now known as the *Medical Mile*. It was not long after this move that Burrell initiated an agreement with Cox Medical Center for inpatient services.

Services for youth with a severe emotional disturbance were added in the same year. The Burrell Foundation was established in 1987 and began its support for service innovation and research. Over the next 15 years, the Burrell Center added new services and new sites, while promoting research and education efforts. When services at Nevada and Fulton State Hospitals and Mid-MO were curtailed in the early 1990s, persons served by these state facilities were successfully reintegrated into their home communities through Burrell's new therapeutic and support programs.

In 1994, Burrell formally affiliated with the 9,000 employee Cox Health Systems and expanded its services beyond its DMH service area of Christian, Dallas, Greene, Polk, Stone, Taney and Webster counties. Through this affiliation, Burrell assumed management of the Cox Center for Addictions, inpatient psychiatry, and hospital-based psychological services and it began the systematic integration of health and behavioral health services. Since then, Burrell has continued to ambitiously position its services in the mainstream of publicly and privately financed health services, now preparing to build a Center for Child and Adolescent Development to better meet the needs of tomorrow.

Burrell Behavioral Health currently provides a broad range of prevention, outpatient, day treatment, supported living, residential, home-based, inpatient, medical clinic-based, outreach, education and research services. Burrell now serves 17,000 persons a year directly and through managed affiliated services at 25 sites. It oversees a staff of 700 clinical and administrative staff, who are supported by an annual budget of $36 million.

Family Guidance Center for Behavioral Healthcare

When Arthur Center opened as the East Central Missouri CMHC in 1967, it had the distinction of having a traditional state mental hospital – Fulton State Hospital – in its catchment area. When Family Guidance Center was awarded its federal CMHC staffing grant in 1978, it had a traditional state mental hospital – St. Joseph State Hospital – down the street. However, by then Family

Guidance had been down the street from "St. Joe" state hospital for more than 15 years. Family Guidance Center was formed when the local Family and Children's Service, Sheltering Arms Guidance Center and the United Cerebral Palsy Developmental Center merged in 1962. Early programs included individual and family counseling, child psychiatry, developmental services to handicapped pre-schoolers, and adoption and foster home care. An annual budget of $95,000 supported services to about 170 individuals.

A CMHC planning grant awarded in 1976 was followed by a staffing grant two years later. Services were expanded under this eight-year federal grant to include inpatient and partial hospitalization, consultation and education, a geriatric program and 24-hour emergency care. The next year brought DMH funding for psychiatric services. In 1988, Family Guidance Center became the DMH administrative agent for the northwest region of Missouri. In 1990, a transitional living program was added to help those with serious mental illness in their adjustment to independence in the community. In 1991, the St. Joseph State Hospital outpatient clinic was transferred to Family Guidance Center, which also opened a psychosocial rehabilitation center.

Since 1986, Family Guidance Center has been a significant provider of treatment services for children who suffer serious emotional and behavioral problems. Services include child and family assessments, day treatment services, in-home and office-based therapy and counseling, parent aids, and family life education. A special program provides skill development to foster families who have agreed to accept in their homes children with an emotional and/or behavioral disturbance.

A premier provider of substance abuse services since 1975, Family Guidance now offers a wide range of services, including residential treatment and services for individuals suffering from a dual diagnosis, as well as specialty interventions for traffic offenders and those with compulsive gambling problems. A pioneer in the area of services for persons in the custody of the Missouri Department of Corrections, Family Guidance's substance abuse treatment services for offenders include the *12-step* self-help approach to treatment as well as cognitive restructuring therapy that helps offenders understand the connection between thoughts and behavior. Residential treatment for offenders also makes use of a modified therapeutic community treatment approach, addressing both substance abuse and the context in which it occurs.

Today, Family Guidance serves the mental health needs of nine northwest Missouri counties: Andrew, Atchison, Buchanan, Clinton, Dekalb, Gentry, Holt, Nodaway, and Worth. According to CEO Garry Hammond, Family Guidance's annual behavioral health budget of nearly $9 million underwrites services for nearly 1,400 adults who suffer from severe and persistent mental illness, 1,500 children with an emotional disturbance and 1,380 people in need of substance abuse treatment.

Crider Center for Mental Health

Like many of the private federally funded CMHCs that preceded it, Crider Center for Mental Health had its origins in state traveling clinics. Karl Wilson, Ph.D.[41] was a community psychology intern and Bonnie DiFranco a social worker at Malcolm Bliss Mental Health Center in 1974-1975 when they first worked together at the traveling clinic in St. Charles.

In 1979, Wilson returned to St. Charles to direct the Mental Health Council of Lincoln, Warren and St. Charles Counties, which began operations in borrowed space. The next year, services were extended through a merger with the Mental Health Council of Franklin County. This merger provided the origin of the fledgling center's new name: Four County Mental Health.[42] In 1994, the

---

[41] For more information, see the *Missouri First-Person Interviews* with Dr. Karl Wilson (pp. 169-178) and Bonnie DiFranco (pp. 199-207).

[42] According to Wilson [110], he preferred to name the operation *Great Rivers Mental Health Center* to reflect the service area's location at the confluence of the Mississippi and Missouri Rivers. Proving that no good idea went to waste in the Missouri mental health community, when that name was left unused by the Four County board, it was appropriated by DMH for its new St. Louis County community mental health agency. Now, both agencies have new names.

agency was renamed to honor Jane Crider, a founding board member, early board chairwoman and tireless advocate for persons with a mental disability.

The agency was awarded a CMHC staffing grant in early 1981, the last such award made in the nation. When the Mental Health Systems Act was repealed later that year, this grant rolled into the state's federal ADAMH block grant. By the time it became part of DMH's state allocation, the original grant award was substantially reduced. However, it was enough to start school-based prevention and early intervention services. A commitment to school-based services has been one of two hallmarks of this center ever since.

The other hallmark has been mental health interventions in large-scale disasters. In 1982, the agency responded to flooding in its service area with disaster counseling to survivors. Disaster counseling was extended beyond Crider Center's service area when it partnered with neighboring COMTREA to assist the survivors of flooding and dioxin contamination in Times Beach. In 1983, Crider Center spearheaded the first NIMH grant in Missouri for disaster recovery counseling. In all, the Crider Center has been awarded five Federal Emergency Management Agency's (FEMA) disaster recovery counseling grants, more than any other CMHC in the country. It has continued to extend disaster counseling and consulting beyond its service area, from North Dakota to South Carolina.

Crider Center was brought into existence at the precise time that the federal government was withdrawing financial support for new CMHCs and Missouri's DMH was experiencing the first of a series of severe budget cutbacks. While the population in its service area has nearly doubled over the past 25 years, its funding has not kept pace. Despite these challenges, the center maintains a robust program – which includes treatment, vocationally oriented rehabilitation clubhouses patterned after the Fountain House model, employment services, housing, community supports and consumer empowerment – for adults with a serious mental illness.

Children challenged with serious emotional disturbance can live safely at home, progress in school and stay out of trouble through family-oriented wraparound services and the development of local systems of care with the center's many community partners. Individuals and families gain the skills they need to meet life's challenges through mental health promotion and early intervention programs, many presented in conjunction with area schools.

Finally, Crider Center provides crisis intervention and acute psychiatric interventions through Behavioral Health Response (BHR), a joint venture with Hopewell, BJC Behavioral Health (BJC BH) and COMTREA. Another of its active partnerships is with Bridgeway Counseling Services, Inc., one of the state's premier substance abuse treatment agencies.

Forty years after the signing of the CMHC Act, Crider Center, through its dedicated CEO Karl Wilson and staff, continues to prove officials at the old NIMH correct when they approved a CMHC grant for this community and this agency.

COMTREA

Some of Missouri's most successful CMHCs began as something else. In 1973, Jefferson County had few service agencies or alternatives for the legal system. Counseling was expensive and only available by traveling to St. Louis. Alcohol or other drug counseling was practically unavailable at any price. The county needed professional mental health services but did not have the finances to create an agency to provide them. One of the first persons to recognize the need was Magistrate Judge John Anderson. Informal discussions among Anderson, Public Defender "Stu" O'Brien and State Probation and Parole District Supervisor Melvin G. Williams led to the establishment of a not-for-profit corporation which would address the county's most serious need: a halfway house. With the help of attorneys Brent Williams and G. William Weier and Sheriff "Buck" Buerger, Community Treatment Incorporated was created on January 22, 1973. This name was shortened to the first syllables of each word;

in that way, *COMTREA* was created. The group picked Stephen F. Huss as executive director. Huss worked for no pay until the agency became financially viable. O'Brien and Anderson contributed $5 each, instructing Huss to "make it grow."

Grow it did, burned down, and grew again. At first, Probation and Parole and DMH's Division of Alcohol and Drug Abuse funded a halfway house. A fire destroyed COMTREA's building in Festus in 1976, and from the ashes emerged a commitment to create a greater, more comprehensive community mental health center serving Jefferson County. In 1978, COMTREA partnered with St. Louis State Hospital to provide medication services for persons with a mental illness[43]. DMH designated COMTREA as the community mental health center for Jefferson County, and the agency took over the small state hospital outreach center at the county health clinic in Hillsboro.

COMTREA has a long history of being responsive to the needs of disaster survivors, including counseling dioxin and flood survivors in the Times Beach area, along with the Crider Center. By 1986, citizens in Jefferson County added their votes of confidence in COMTREA by approving a local property tax, first set at $800,000 annually. In 2003, that local tax effort yielded $2 million for mental health services in the county [56].

From a halfway house built in 1973 to meet the needs of seventeen local boys who had criminal charges and were drug users, COMTREA grew to become a comprehensive community mental health center. It offers a wide array of services that includes diagnosis, counseling and therapy services; psychiatric rehabilitation services; comprehensive chemical abuse services; domestic violence counseling; case management services to clients; follow-up and aftercare services; day treatment and other specialized services for children; specialized seniors' services; crisis response (flood, other disasters); and more than 100 residential beds for emergency care and ongoing treatment.

---

[43] See also Bonnie DiFranco's *Missouri First Person Interview* [pp. 199-207].

Two $5 donations in 1973 have paid off handsomely for the citizens of Jefferson County. Thirty years later, and still under the direction of Dr. Steve Huss, COMTREA has an annual budget in excess of $9.5 million and operates in seven cities. Its staff of 207 serves more than 5,000 persons a year.

North Central Missouri Mental Health Center

Like COMTREA, the agency that would become the North Central Missouri Mental Health Center was organized to meet the substance abuse prevention and treatment needs of its community. Green Hills Substance Abuse Task Force was incorporated in June 1974 to "develop individual and family counseling, pre-treatment counseling where alcoholism is involved," and to provide educational programs. Its board of directors was comprised of three representatives from each of the nine counties in the Green Hills area: Caldwell, Daviess, Grundy, Harrison, Linn, Livingston, Mercer, Putnam and Sullivan. This number was later reduced. Reverend Larry Linville of Milan served as the first president of the board of directors, Sister Kathleen Reichert of Chillicothe served as the first vice president, and Daniel Evans served as the first secretary and treasurer. Later in its initial year of operation, Dan Kenney assumed the treasurer position.

Initially, the group received a DMH grant for substance abuse services. With the anticipation of funding, the board of directors employed Rex Thompson of St. Joseph to serve as its first paid employee. The agency's first office was a small room in the courthouse, donated by Grundy County. The group struggled through its first three years, often on the verge of financial collapse. Treasurer Kenney periodically made personal loans to secure working capital to pay staff salaries and other expenses.

In 1976, Green Hills began an alcohol-related traffic offenders program for individuals who were charged with drinking and driving. The next summer, the board of directors made the decision to go for "all or nothing" by hiring two full-time staff. The next year, it expanded its services again and changed its name to Green Hills Counseling Service. In 1981 and 1982, Green Hills added outpatient alcohol and drug abuse services and established an apartment program for individuals with serious mental health problems. In 1982, it changed its name to North Central Missouri Mental Health Center.

Over the past 25 years, North Central has expanded its services to include assessment, referral, case management for children and adults, crisis intervention/resolution, individual counseling for children and adults, psychosocial rehabilitation for adults, and psychiatric medication services for children and adults, as well as two residential substance abuse treatment programs. These services are delivered through satellite offices in six of its nine counties. Over the past 25 years, North Central has grown from an annual budget of $28,000 to $1.7 million, with a staff of more than 40 employees, all ably directed by Executive Director Lori Irvine.

Bootheel Counseling Services

One of the greatest assets of the Missouri Coalition of Community Mental Health Centers is the longevity of many of its member CEOs. Two CEOs with remarkable tenure continue to direct adjacent centers in far southeast Missouri: Ron Steinmetz at Bootheel Counseling Services and Myra Callahan at Family Counseling Center.

Bootheel Counseling Services was initially incorporated as Tri County Counseling Center in November 1975. It opened on January 2, 1976, in a converted restaurant that it shared with three other businesses. The center was started as a partnership between the local Tri County MHA and DMH. Previously, this area was served by a one-person outreach office and monthly traveling clinics from Farmington State Hospital (now Southeast Missouri Mental Health Center) held at churches in Scott, Stoddard and Mississippi counties. In 1975, members of the local MHA met with then DMH Director Dr. Harold Robb to request more mental health services for the three-county area. Attending that meeting was a social worker from the DMH-run Sikeston Regional Center for the Developmentally Disabled. Robb made this commitment: he would provide with state funds a social worker as executive director, the nurse therapist from the outreach office, and an alcohol and drug counselor, if the MHA would incorporate, hire a secretary, fund an office, and work toward providing additional services in the future. The social worker from the regional center was transferred to the payroll of Farmington State Hospital and was assigned as the executive director of the new private, not-for-profit corporation. He remained a state employee until the center's board hired him six years later.

During its early years, the center's services consisted of counseling for a wide range of problems, providing follow-up to persons with a serious mental illness who were seen in the traveling clinics, and community education. Much emphasis was placed on working with clients in groups. The budget in those early years was under $100,000, with a staff of four. When New Madrid County was added to the service area in 1982, the center's name was changed to Bootheel Mental Health Center. The name was changed again in 1991 to Bootheel Counseling Services. A full-time branch office was established in Stoddard County in 1983. A separate psychosocial rehabilitation facility was built in 1992, and in 1997, an 18,000-square-foot facility was built to consolidate programs and staff who had been distributed across different locations.

Many things have changed at Bootheel Counseling Services since the MHA representatives first met with Dr. Robb. The center now has a staff of 67. Its current budget is in excess of $3 million, allowing its staff to be more proactive in their treatment of adults who suffer from a serious mental illness and of children who have a severe emotional disturbance. One thing remains the same, however. The soft-spoken, dedicated and forward-thinking regional center social worker who attended that meeting 28 years ago, who served as the young CMHC's executive director while a Farmington State Hospital employee, and was later hired by the center in the same role, is still there. He is Ron Steinmetz.

Family Counseling Center

Go to the southeastern tip of Missouri, where it forms an apostrophe separating Arkansas and Tennessee. Follow the Arkansas border west from Pemiscot and Dunklin counties to the point where Ripley and Oregon counties meet. If you go north from Butler and Ripley to Carter, Wayne and Reynolds counties, you are in the mental health service area of Family Counseling Center. At the center's headquarters in Kennett, you will meet its executive director, Myra Callahan. She has worked there for more than 25 years.

If you had visited there in 1977, you would have met her then, but in the role of administrative assistant. Years of perseverance and scores of weekend roundtrips to college in Columbia led to a bachelor's degree for Myra in 1989. Three years later, she was certified as a substance abuse counselor, and in 1993 she was awarded a master of science in administration degree by Southeast Missouri State University in Cape Girardeau. Her career at Family Counseling followed the same trajectory: first hired as administrative assistant, then named director of day treatment, then administrator and later executive director, a post she has held for more than 20 years.

In many ways, the history of Family Counseling Center resembles Myra's personal history. It was founded in 1976 as a small substance abuse treatment program. The next year, Dunklin County arranged to repay part of a federal CMHC grant that had not become fully operational by making the first in a series of annual grants to the center for mental health services. Building on a monthly traveling clinic headed by the eminent Dr. Emmett Hoctor of Farmington State Hospital, many of the early services provided by the traveling clinic were continued on a daily basis by the first Kennett unit.

Today, Family Counseling Center's staff of 200 offers a full range of programs to the 5,100 persons they serve annually. These programs include intensive case management, psychiatric rehabilitation, substance abuse treatment and rehabilitation, residential substance abuse treatment, prevention and outpatient services. For more than 20 years, Myra Callahan has successfully guided Family Counseling Center and its staff of 200 dedicated employees to its current level of prominence and annual budget of $8 million.

Ozarks Medical Center - Behavioral Healthcare

Keep traveling west, and you will come to Oregon, Shannon, Texas, Howell, Wright, Douglas and Ozark counties, the service area for Ozarks Medical Center (OMC), headquartered in West Plains. The newest of the community mental health agencies in Missouri, OMC was awarded the designation as administrative agent for DMH in 1997, replacing Ozark Area Care and Counseling, a mental health agency with deep roots in this rural part of Missouri.

Their story begins in 1978, when a group of concerned citizens under the guidance of Colin Collins founded Community Care and Counseling (CCC) in West Plains, Missouri. The mission of CCC was to provide access to mental health services for residents of rural Missouri. Simultaneously in Houston, Missouri, local citizens started another community mental health agency called Ozark Area Care and Counseling (OACC). DMH provided funding for mental health services to both organizations, as well as outreach workers from Farmington State Hospital; Mike Newton was assigned the West Plains area and Alan Leak worked in Houston. Ann Dugan, founder of Studio 410, was also awarded a POS contract by DMH and established a day treatment program to assist adults with chronic mental illness to develop increased social skills to live more productive, independent and self-directed lives.

In the early 1980s CCC, OACC and Studio 410 merged under the OACC name. In 1987, the developing OACC struggled to maintain financial viability. OMC, a local community-owned hospital, agreed to provide administrative management services for OACC until that organization could stabilize its financial situation. In 1989, OMC returned management of OACC to an independent board.

In 1991, OMC began to expand outpatient mental health services through a network of rural health clinics it owned and operated. Carlissa Gilliam, OMC director of mental health services, was named to oversee the clinical and administrative aspects of this program expansion. When DMH designated OMC as the administrative agent for DMH service area 18 in 1997, it led to a consolidation of inpatient and comprehensive outpatient services, streamlining continuity of care for a large number of mental health consumers. Approximately 750 consumers made the transition and Ozarks Medical Center-Behavioral Healthcare (OMC-BHC) became a reality.

Services are currently delivered in facilities in West Plains and Mountain Grove. OMC-BHC serves an average of 7,000 clients annually through its network of rural health clinics, successfully pairing comprehensive mental health care with primary care to meet the growing needs of the rural population. The consumers of OMC-BHC's psychosocial rehabilitation program run a catering business that serves the medical center and area organizations, and they operate a business that shreds confidential medical information. Consumers also create and distribute a daily newsletter and operate a snack bar at the West Plains center. A preschool program operates in West Plains and provides intensive treatment to children ages 3 to 6 who are diagnosed with serious emotional disorders. Community-based case management serves an average of 300 adults with a serious and persistent mental illness. The medical staff consists of four full-time psychiatrists who specialize in child, adult and forensic psychiatry and addictions. The staff of 85 also includes advance practice nurses, clinical psychologists, licensed social workers and counselors.

Clark Community Mental Health Center

Begun as the Barry-Lawrence County Counseling Service in 1971, this center was first organized and staffed by clinicians moonlighting from the Ozark Community Mental Health Center. Encouraged by Cravens at the Division of Mental Diseases and supported by a small grant, Frank Compton (now the Clark Center executive director) and his Ozark colleagues worked on their days off because, according to Compton [17], "We were excited about delivering mental health services in rural Missouri." This unique outreach effort led to the establishment of the program headquartered in Monett. In 1989, the agency's name was changed to honor Tom Clark, the president of the board who had been killed in a motorcycle accident, along with his wife.

The Clark Center has progressed from its early beginnings as an outpatient counseling center to being the sole provider of services for the people who have the most severe and persistent mental illnesses and for those who have the most severe substance abuse problems, in Dade, Barry and Lawrence counties. Despite its size, the Clark Center has maintained an outpatient treatment program that balances the needs of persons with acute and persistent mental illnesses. The center has 65 employees and a $2.6 million dollar annual budget. Services, including psychosocial rehabilitation, case management, medication services, crisis intervention[44], and special programs for children and families, are provided each year to 2,000 consumers.

Pathways Community Behavioral Healthcare

An innovative solution to the challenges of providing high-quality, accessible and affordable mental health services began to take shape in west central Missouri in the late 1990s. Over the past several years, the leadership and staff members of the five independent mental health agencies profiled below have forged Pathways Community Behavioral Healthcare, Inc., a grand organization of more than 530 staff serving the mental health needs of Missourians in 21 counties.[45] Forming a broad belt of counties nearly across Missouri's mid-section, from Cuba, Missouri, at the

---

[44] In his *Missouri First-Person Interview*, Dr. Morty Lebedun [pp. 133-141] describes his observations on Clark Center's disaster intervention program.

[45] Through its combined mental health and substance abuse programs, Pathways serves 32 counties with a total population of more than 1.1 million Missourians, nearly one-fifth of the citizens in the state.

east and the Kansas border at the west, Pathways operates at 26 office locations, providing over 20 different programs and services ranging from prevention and education to intervention and treatment.

The roots of Pathways, however, go back more than 30 years, when concern about the lack of resources for addressing substance abuse needs in Henry, Bates and St. Clair counties led to the establishment of Community Counseling Consultants (CCC). In 1974, CCC began operating as a not-for-profit community agency for a total of nine counties: the original three, plus Vernon, Pettis, Benton, Cedar, Hickory and Morgan. Approximately ten employees provided outpatient treatment for substance abuse out of a small "office" in the basement of a home on Highway 7 west of Clinton, Missouri. In the early 1980s, the demand for more services portended the need for a larger, more efficient building, with adolescent and adult residential treatment units. In 1987, Jerry Osborn was named CEO, and he raised over $350,000 for such a facility, which was completed in 1992.

In his *Missouri First-Person Interview*, Osborn [pp. 217-221], details how managed care and changes in the mental health field caused CCC to evaluate its options for survival. A strategic plan was developed to address issues that would keep CCC a viable provider for community-based services. In March 1997, CCC joined with West Central Missouri Mental Health Center in Warrensburg, Missouri. A new agency, Pathways Community Behavioral Healthcare, emerged with the same mission – to provide comprehensive, high-quality, accessible and affordable behavioral healthcare to Missourians – while encouraging the personal and professional growth of its staff members.

West Central Missouri Mental Health Center

West Central Missouri Mental Health Center was formed in May 1970 to provide a full-time clinic for mental health services in Johnson, Lafayette, and Cass counties. Prior to then, a physician from Western MO in Kansas City staffed an outreach clinic in Warrensburg two days each month. At that time, West Central's board of directors generated funds to establish a clinic in space donated by Johnson County Memorial Hospital in Warrensburg. Through the years preceding its merger with CCC, West Central expanded its outpatient offerings with a day treatment program and a residential substance abuse treatment program. It also opened a satellite office in Harrisonville.

Southwest Missouri Mental Health Center

Additional opportunities to provide accessible services evolved in July 1998 when Pathways was awarded a DMH contract to provide outpatient services in the southwest region of Missouri. Services in this area had been provided by an agency known as Southwest Missouri Mental Health Center, which was created following the closing of the Nevada State Hospital. Under this contract, Pathways assumed responsibility for clinical offices in Nevada and El Dorado Springs and has subsequently established services in Butler.

Family Mental Health Center

In Jefferson City, Missouri's capital city, local citizens concerned about the need for children's mental health services established the Cole County Mental Health Services clinic, staffed by outreach workers from Fulton State Hospital. When the administrative agent system was established in 1981, the Cole County program was designated to oversee community mental health programs in its county as well as in Miller, Osage, Laclede, Camden and Pulaski counties, and the agency was renamed Family Mental Health Center. Clinicians from Fulton State Hospital who staffed the mental health clinics in these counties were reassigned to positions back at the hospital, and general revenue funding was made available to provide clinical, administrative and support staff.

Family Mental Health's expanded area of administrative responsibility included the independent La Cam Counseling Center. Established in 1974, La Cam provided services in Laclede and Camden counties in conjunction with clinicians assigned by Fulton State Hospital. In 1984, La Cam changed its name to Northern

Ozarks. It merged with Family Mental Health Center in 1990 when the comprehensive psychosocial rehabilitation program was introduced in Missouri. Family Mental Health Center merged with Pathways Community Behavioral Healthcare, Inc. in July 1998.

FOCUS (Family Oriented Counseling Services)

Community mental health services began in Rolla and surrounding counties in 1973 when the Rolla Area Counseling Clinic was incorporated to provide follow-up care for patients released from Farmington State Hospital. Changing its name to Central Ozarks Mental Health Center in 1978, the center expanded programming to include supportive services, day treatment and psychiatry. In the early 1990s, the focus changed as the CPR model was developed for improving the care given to adults with chronic and severe mental illnesses. In 1993, the agency's name changed again to FOCUS: Family Oriented Counseling Services. In 1996, FOCUS was awarded the DMH contract for mental health services for Gasconade County. In 1999, the FOCUS board merged the agency serving Phelps, Crawford, Dent and Maries counties into Pathways Community Behavioral Healthcare.

Dr. Dick Cravens was affiliated with his home state's mental health program from late 1959 to early 1976. He held many posts in Missouri, primarily associated with developing community mental health centers throughout the state. A psychologist by training, Dr. Cravens served as Missouri's director of community mental health. His service in Missouri was followed by an equally distinguished career in the federal government. In 1992, Dr. Cravens retired from his position as director of refugee health, Office of the Assistant Secretary for Health, U.S. Department of Health and Human Services.

In the early 1960s, it was my job to contact and to meet with representatives of the communities – the Shirley Fearons of Missouri – to start consulting with them and to determine the interest and needs of the community with respect to mental health issues. When I first joined the Department of Mental Health, I did a lot of work with the state hospitals and got to know a lot of community providers. I spoke often at PTA meetings and other community gatherings about the possibility of having a mental health facility in their community. There were times when I would give 30 talks a week, beating the bushes all over Missouri. I would meet with any group that was interested in the community mental health center movement. I also had access to communities through legislators. For example, Senator Al Spradling was the first person to put me in touch with people in Cape Girardeau. He was a mental health advocate and a staunch supporter of the division

In Mexico there were three people with whom I met: a local physician; Colonel Stribling, who owned Mexico Military Academy; and Bob White, who owned and published the newspaper. All three were influential in that community; they were prominent socially and they had a say in what happened in Mexico. I met with them often and they were the ones who made the decision to go ahead with development of the mental health center and to tie it to the hospital. They wanted community-based services and provided the local leadership that is vital in an initiative of this sort. That was the interest of all community representatives – to make services available, to be responsible for them and to locate them in their communities.

The contact I worked most with in Joplin was a person I first met at Nevada State Hospital, where he was a social worker. I recall that there was a Nevada State Hospital traveling clinic in Joplin, and this operation underscored the interest in and need for a community mental health center.

The sparkplug in Springfield was Probate Court Judge Don Burrell. At one time, he was a member of the state mental health commission. He had some mental health insight and sensitivity, and he and I hit it off personally, as friends. Don was the driving force in Springfield and wanted a mental health center there. He also had access to contacts and to money. That was a relatively straightforward and easy operation to bring into place. They started off as a freestanding center and were located in a multi-story building downtown. There was an arrangement with one of the local hospitals for inpatient services, but all their other services were housed in this multistory building. Their first director was Dr. Todd Schaible, who was very innovative and very sensitive to the fiscal needs of the center and who found ways to pay for the whole program. He was very, very good. As an aside, quite frequently there was a current of resistance from private practitioners. This was particularly true in Springfield, where there was a large private practice community.

Shirley Fearon got things going in south Jackson County. She was so good; if you had a dozen people like her in the state you could have accomplished so much. She was a bird dog. She never gave up, and when we would encounter disappointments, she would find ways to go over, under or around. She was superb in identifying the needs of the community and mobilizing resources.

After leaving Mexico where he was the center director, Jack Viar went to North Kansas City, where he became director of that local community mental health center and contributed so much to the development of the movement in Missouri.

I spent a great deal of time with representatives in Independence and Hannibal. There was also interest in a community mental health center in St. Joseph, but at that time, the local leadership was missing. It may have been that the presence of the St. Joseph State Hospital masked the need for a CMHC.

Some of the early applicants for community mental health center grants were hospitals, and they were tuned to operating costs. These people had a good understanding of fiscal issues and were further along when it came to supporting services. In contrast, mental health people were used to working in not-for-profit agencies where somebody else paid the bills. They were not sophisticated in the money part of the operation, and I thought that in the beginning this was a weak part of the program: "How are you going to pay for this when the federal money runs out?"

I had a lot of dealings with the Kirksville School of Osteopathy, too. There was a great deal of interest in developing and operating a community mental health center, but the necessary resources were not available at that time.

As far as Malcolm Bliss and Western MO were concerned, when they came into the Department of Mental Health, they were so far ahead of what everyone else was doing in terms of services provided, philosophy, sophistication and quality of personnel. The three contacts at Western Missouri were Drs. Bob Barnes, Charlie Wilkinson and Robijn Hornstra. They were marvelous representatives of the community mental health movement. Western Missouri actually served as a prototype for the federal government in the CMHC construction and staffing grant programs. Dr. George Ulett, later director of the Missouri Division of Mental Diseases, was director of Malcolm Bliss and responsible for the quality and direction of the program there.

There were some sticking points in the development of community mental health centers. Sometimes it was difficult for the disciplines to work together because the pecking order was still pretty strong among psychiatry, psychology and social work. Nurses were also becoming more active in the community mental health field. We always worked together, but there was still an awareness of the pecking order. I think things are much better today than they were then. It was difficult then for psychiatry to accept a social worker or a psychologist as a center director. I don't know that there was ever a problem in practice, but initially there was resistance.

When I first went to Missouri, the state hospitals were more or less in the warehousing mode. There was treatment, to be sure, but there was also a very large chronic inpatient population. This was due, in part, to the limitations of treatment strategies available at that time. State hospitals were communities unto themselves, separate communities from the larger community. Relationships between the state hospitals and the CMHCs were never really good, in part because the state hospitals were threatened by the CMHCs. They were new; they were shiny. The people were generally better paid. They had a different point of view and philosophy of dealing with the mentally ill.

One of the things I worked on very hard was to have a formal relationship between the state hospitals and the CMHCs for purposes of referral, follow-up and aftercare. I was never successful. The state hospitals did not want to give up responsibility for patients. It was never a very happy relationship between the state hospitals and the CMHCs. Some of the things said by Dr. Felix and others just prior to the CMHC Act, about the goal being to shut down the state hospitals, were unfortunate things to say. I used to argue that there must be a place for the chronically mentally ill, a place to shelter and care for people who had reached maximum treatment benefits and required a protected living and working environment.

RESPONSIBILITY FOR A SPECIFIED POPULATION: That was the catchment area; it was never an issue, as I recall. People were aware that they had to extend themselves out into the surrounding geography and provide services. This was so important in the large rural areas of Missouri.

PREVENTION AND EARLY INTERVENTION: These were concepts at that time that were still pretty new. They were foreign to many practitioners. There was general interest, but the techniques for prevention and early intervention were really not well understood, developed or disseminated. Consultation services were not well understood and probably not provided to the extent intended by the CMHC Act. This is understandable because as a technique it was not generally taught or practiced by mental health professionals. It simply wasn't used much.

TREATING PEOPLE IN THEIR HOME COMMUNITIES: This was very important; in fact, it was one of my strong selling points. Treat people here in the community. If hospitalization is required, do so quickly and discharge the patient as soon as maximum inpatient treatment benefits are realized. Do not prolong hospitalization. Early identification and intervention were valuable tools for decreasing and shortening the length of inpatient hospitalization.

CONTINUUM OF CARE: Continuity of care was a new concept for people and it was something that kind of puzzled them. I don't know why it was such a difficult issue, but it had to be explained carefully and in detail. It was something where you could always see a question mark over the heads of the people with whom I was consulting, and I don't know why. It departed from traditional training and experience. Partial hospitalization, one of the required services, was difficult to design and put into operation. At the time, it was new to many mental health professionals and it was so different from the traditional and familiar programs of outpatient and inpatient care.

LINKAGES WITH OTHER ORGANIZATIONS: Linkages with other community agencies was a concept that many mental health professionals were not accustomed to and did not understand. Over a period of time, it was accepted.

FISCAL AND PROGRAMMATIC ACCOUNTABILITY: This was a stumbling block for many mental health people because they really did not understand fiscal issues and program evaluation. Many professionals would say, "I'm not concerned with the money. I don't have to worry about the money." I would talk with them about charging fees, but they were very uncomfortable about money and fees. The perspective is different for the private practitioner. It was something I hammered home: "Pretty soon you're going to have to pay for this. You'll have to start thinking about this."

CITIZEN PARTICIPATION: Citizen participation probably was the key to the whole thing. I'm not sure that community mental health centers would be the success they are today without local involvement in the centers' inception and operation.

If there had not been a federal program, I believe that the state would have put in some community-based services, but nowhere to the extent of what was developed with the federal program. The programs would have probably consisted of traditional outpatient services and consequently been limited in effectiveness.

MISSOURI FIRST-PERSON INTERVIEW WITH:

JACK VIAR

Jack Viar completed the graduate social work program at the University of Missouri in 1964. From 1964 through 1967, he held a variety of positions at Fulton State Hospital. In 1967, Mr. Viar was hired as the director of Missouri's first not-for-profit CMHC in Mexico, Missouri.

From 1976 to 1981, he directed the Tri-County Mental Health Center in North Kansas City, Missouri. He was a founder of the Missouri Coalition of Community Mental Health Centers, and the Metro Council of CMHCs, and he held various posts with the National Council of CMHCs. From 1981 to 2000, Jack Viar was in private practice in the Kansas City area. During this period, he was an active consultant both to the Missouri DMH and other CMHCs.

I did my block placement in graduate school at Fulton State Hospital and stayed for three years after my graduation in 1964. You could try new things there and the administration was supportive. I remember when family therapy first came out and I thought that Virginia Satir and that whole Palo Alto group were the answer to everything. At Fulton, you could try things like that. I worked in the Biggs forensic unit and in the youth center. In my last year, I was supervisor of adult services at the clinic in the acute section. With all three patient population groups I had the opportunity to try new therapy approaches. It was an invaluable learning experience for me.

Fulton used to send a person up to Mexico once a week to facilitate a child guidance clinic at Audrain Hospital. When I was at the Fulton youth center, I was the person who went up. I had gotten acquainted with Woody Lee, who was the hospital administrator at Audrain County Hospital. Woody had made a couple of attempts to get a CMHC construction grant, and unfortunately, they had been rejected. A part of that was simply that he was not a *mental healther*; he did not use mental health terms and wasn't particularly familiar with mental health programs. He asked me to come up in the evening after work for a while and rewrite the construction grant application. I did that, and the grant was awarded to Audrain. That eventually led to an offer to become the hospital's director of mental health services.

One of the interesting things is that they offered me $12,000, and my wife was embarrassed to tell her folks that I was going to earn that much money. For the state, I was making about $8,000, and that was good money. When I worked for the state, it was the opposite of what has been going on recently: I got two or three raises a year. I certainly had no complaints. In fact, I thought it was pretty good. The hospital in Mexico purchased a little bungalow across the street and refurbished it. We worked out of that little house for about a year and a half during the construction phase. Colonel Stribling was the chairman of the board of the hospital. Bob White was a mover and shaker in Mexico, as was Dr. Ed Wallace.

There was beginning to be some attention to the idea that the state hospital was not the best alternative and that the idea of out-of-sight, out-of-mind was really not appropriate. The idea was to treat people in their home community. It was not to build a small state hospital; it was quite the opposite. If you had chronic patients, you had the state hospital as a back-up. The idea was to provide a more acute focus.

The scary part for me was that there was no model. There was nobody to talk with about whether this would work or that would work. You only had what you read in books and journal articles. The staffing grant gave us a lot of freedom to assemble the staff. The biggest obstacle to building a staff was attracting a psychiatrist to come over there. I went to a couple of national meetings to try to recruit psychiatrists. The first guy I got came from the state hospital in Cherokee, Iowa. He was with us about a year and a half before he developed some health problems. We had a contract with several psychiatrists from Mid-MO. Finally, we recruited Zaki Ajans full time. That was a huge deal. I just think the world of Zaki. He is a hard worker and a great guy. He had a residency in internal medicine as well as psychiatry. He had the whole ball of wax, and he just was very pleasant to work with.

In North Kansas City, the hospital already had a construction and a staffing grant. Dave Wiebe and Hal Boyts, social workers in Johnson County, Kansas, helped hospital administrator Charlie Clausen do some of the grant work, like develop the staffing pattern and things that a non-*mental-healther* would not be familiar with. So a lot of that was done when I got there. They hadn't broken ground yet, and the hospital leased a suite of offices in the professional building across the street for us. That was our base of operations. It was another program that I was very proud of.

That center was a little more fiscally responsible for several reasons. First, as I got a little more experience and knowledge, I began to realize that mental health needed to pay its own way and not ride on the coattails of the other hospital departments. So I made a much more concerted effort to bring it to a break-even point than I did in Mexico. In Mexico, I was so naïve that I thought, "Well, the hospital wanted this, so why are they complaining that we are losing so much money?" I never completely tied those two things together in Mexico; in North Kansas City, I did. I had a much different emphasis with the staff. For example, I would say, "You can't have no-shows and think that's a good deal because you get an hour free. That kind of mentality has to change and you have to do things to minimize no-shows and things like that." We came much closer to breaking even, and running a deficit was a bit of a sore point with some people, like the finance officer at the hospital.

When a new administrator arrived, he pretty well cleaned house in the hospital. Profit became a big issue. He systematically released all the assistant administrators and people at my level, except me. We were pretty much on opposite philosophical tracks. I think the reason he didn't get rid of me was that the tax levy drive was just getting underway, and it would have been pretty disruptive to that effort to get rid of the director of mental health in the middle of that. And then the tax levy was successful, and it would have been a poor time to get rid of the director amid all the positive publicity about the center and what it was doing for the citizens. That protected me for maybe a year after the tax levy was passed.

Charlie Clausen, the hospital administrator who hired me at North Kansas City, had a pretty much hands-off approach to dealing with me. From the beginning, that was a fairly vibrant facility, with lots of enthusiasm. The new administrator, however, was very conservative financially and would give me ultimatums. That was when the concept of community outreach and the whole concept of involving the citizens began to disintegrate at the hospital.

RESPONSIBILITY FOR A SPECIFIED POPULATION: Prior to the mental health centers, I think the hospitals at both Mexico and North Kansas City were a little more constricted with regard to the areas they served. Because of the population requirements and the designation of a catchment area, the hospitals began to reach out to a much larger community. Twenty years ago, North Kansas City Hospital was a relatively small local hospital. The mental health center was sort of the beginning of its expansion. In both facilities, the treatment concept was simply enlarged.

PREVENTION AND EARLY INTERVENTION: Prevention and outreach were incorporated into the medical model. In a rural setting it was more difficult to do prevention, but it was more essential because we had a catchment area that was geographically much larger. The whole notion of hiring somebody to do just consultation and education was pretty foreign, and was looked at pretty skeptically by people. Consultation was more nebulous. How did you know if you were helping anyone?

TREATING PEOPLE IN THEIR HOME COMMUNITIES: Providing mental health treatment in the community was a relatively new concept. There was a skepticism about anybody going into any sort of mental hospital, especially a state hospital. At Mexico, it was generally more accepted than having to travel down to Fulton 30 miles away. Fulton had a 100-year history and much of that was mysterious and scary to ordinary citizens.

I think the physicians really welcomed the concept that somebody that they were treating in their practice for a medical problem but who was also experiencing psychological problems might be hospitalized right there. The doctors had the same suspicions about the state hospitals that everybody else did. The way our program was promoted was that the family physician was going to be an integral part of the treatment team, and we were not going to take their patients away from them. We encouraged them to follow their patients on the psychiatric unit, and they welcomed that. Because Zaki had a residency in internal medicine, as well as in psychiatry, he was really respected. Everybody who dealt with Zaki respected him.

CONTINUUM OF CARE: The beauty of the CMHC, as opposed to the state hospital, was the continuity of treatment. You could see people initially as an outpatient, and if they did deteriorate, then you had a partial hospitalization program and if they further deteriorated, you had an inpatient program. Because all of this was in place, that's exactly what you did. We also had greater access to the patients' families. That was more advantageous than sending somebody 40 or 50 miles away even for outpatient services. People simply wouldn't travel that far.

Another problem in a rural area was the partial hospitalization program. You can't reasonably expect a family to drive 50 miles every day to come into a partial hospital program. And even though we encouraged that, it just never really got off the ground in Mexico. It was so much different in North Kansas City where we had a much greater population base within 10 miles of the center and it was reasonable to put an emphasis on that.

MULTIDISCIPLINARY TEAMS: Two things we initiated in Mexico proved fairly successful. We had an African-American nurse's aide whom we trained in consultation, who worked with the Head Start program and the elementary schools. She was an important link to the African-American community. Also, one of the nurses was married to a Baptist minister. As you know, in a small rural community, the Baptist minister in the African-American community is a pretty well-respected guy. She was a really neat lady and she gave us a lot of credibility. That tied us to that part of the community. They both did a lot to pave the way for us.

There were probably six or eight clinical staff, and each of us included a nurse in all the clinical stuff that we did. The objective was to give that nurse sufficient experience and supervision so that she could operate independently in an outpatient or partial hospitalization setting. They were very effective. They led groups and were co-therapists in family therapy. They were an important part of the clinical team.

LINKAGES WITH OTHER ORGANIZATIONS: In Mexico, there weren't a whole lot of other social service agencies. We did work closely with the juvenile office, child welfare and the school system. In North Kansas City, we established the Metro Council of mental health agencies in the Kansas City area with Shirley Fearon and Jim McKee and Brenda Pelofsky. We started a sexual abuse network north of the river that included all of the agencies serving children and therapists who worked with sexually abused kids. It was educational and provided an opportunity to liaison with other child advocates.

FISCAL AND PROGRAMMATIC ACCOUNTABILITY: In Mexico, money was always an issue. I remember the mental health center certainly did not make money, and around budget time we would be asking for more staff or a new car or something like that and that was a pretty uncomfortable process. I was so naïve and didn't give sufficient attention to dealing with it as a business, while in North Kansas City it was really impressed upon me, and I began to realize the program was going to be tied to revenue. If I didn't begin to generate some bucks, I couldn't continue to ask for program expansion money in the budget for continuing education and other things that were non-revenue producing.

Toward the latter part of my tenure at Mexico, we started the ball rolling on the Missouri Coalition of Community Mental Health Centers. I think that at that time, the main reason that the Coalition was formed was the belief that community mental health needed a collective voice. I couldn't go down to Jefferson City with any kind of clout, nor could another center director. But if we could go together, if we could present a collective request, then we would be more effective than if we lobbied separately. I don't think the department ever thought, "Who are those upstarts who are trying to take our business away?" Dick Cravens was very helpful. He represented the department, but he was very supportive of the community mental health concept. The department forwarded 314 (d) money to us and they were helpful in many more ways. If it wasn't for the department, the CMHCs would not have gotten off the ground, and a lot of that was due to Dick Cravens.

Morty Lebedun, reared in St. Louis, has remained committed to Missouri throughout his career. After earning degrees in psychology, social work and sociology, Dr. Lebedun experienced the Missouri community mental health movement first-hand. He has directed three community mental health centers and has also served as the director of community psychiatry for the state Department of Mental Health. He served as the chair of the Missouri Coalition of Community Mental Health Centers, remaining active in that organization for 25 years.

For many years, Dr. Lebedun has enjoyed teaching classes at various colleges and universities. He has a creative ability to hold opposing points of view on nearly any subject, and he truly believes in the forces that have created and supported community mental health.

I started my professional career in 1967 at Fulton State Hospital, as a clinical casework assistant. After six months in that facility, I was fortunate to be able to transfer my work-study program to Mid-Missouri Mental Health Center in Columbia, Missouri. We were a bunch of young, energetic, idealistic staff who were just entering or who were completing graduate school. It was an exciting place for me to complete my MSW work.

I then returned to graduate school at Mizzou, pursuing my doctoral degree in medical sociology and leaving Columbia in 1973. I was hired by Jack Viar in June of that year to work for Tri-County Community Mental Health Center, which wasn't operational until later that year. We were in temporary space in the professional building on the campus with the North Kansas City Hospital. The construction work was completed on the facility and it officially opened in October 1973. I remained at Tri-County until 1976 when I joined St. Francis Mental Health Center in Cape Girardeau.

Lou Masterman had just retired and the mental health program was moving into the new St. Francis Medical Center.

Mental health was reborn in that environment, because for the first time there was a dedicated 20-bed inpatient unit, with all the outpatient offices on the first floor. In 1976, I wrote an operations grant that allowed us to develop the twelve required services. We added another 20 staff or so. Since then, the medical center constructed a 20,000-square-foot freestanding facility. The hospital paid back federal construction money which was then used to build the new center.

Many of the programs and services at St. Francis worked well for that community, that area. However, we always had concerns about funding. We knew the federal dollars were on an eight-year declining share of operations cost which made everybody mindful of the pending deficit if new revenue was not found. That was a big motivator. When the state mill tax legislation was changed in 1978 to allow individual counties to pass a mental health tax, our funding world changed for the better. Fortunately, Perry, Ste. Genevieve and Cape Girardeau counties passed the tax. I think the mill tax contributed close to 30% - 40% of the operating capital for the agency by 1982. It was essential funding when the block grants resulted in reduced federal support.

St. Francis CMHC was noted for its strong consultation and education component. The center spent significant time and effort on prevention. We worked closely with the schools and we hired a school counselor as a prevention coordinator. The success of the educational programs garnered support for the tax campaigns.

In June 1982, I left St. Francis to join DMH as the director of community psychiatry. The duties of the new position included managing block grants for the CMHCs. I worked with Dorn Schuffman to develop per capita funding plans. These early efforts by central office involved collaboration to equitably distribute CMHC funds statewide.

In the 1980s, the department's commitment to treating people with a serious mental illness, and the expansion of the CPR program, brought needed change. The CPR program, with its focus on serious and persistent mental illness, caused some hospitals to ultimately close their community behavioral health service. I think the hospitals perceived that patients with a serious mental illness were not a good mix with their acute care populations.

During the 1980s, the Coalition of Community Mental Health Centers became more active in bringing people together as advocates for the system. Kathy Carter was hired in 1979. Prior to that event, the Coalition included members Jack Viar, Jim McKee, Ken Foster and several other people coming to Jeff City to share program ideas. It was not a functional entity from a political point of view. With Kathy's arrival, and the block grants following, we really cemented the idea that we must work as a total system. There were service areas to address needs of defined populations. The idea of all the agencies pulling together for a common purpose became reality. The Coalition galvanized that and created a forum where best practices could be talked about. I remember the early days of the Coalition being a time when we discussed programs and treatment approaches.

In those days, the focus was on building program capacity and certainly when Paul Ahr served as DMH director, he placed a focus on levels of care and the funding to make it happen. Ironically, it became a time to expand programming, to take small programs and actually move them up to the next level of responsibility. It did allow people to look at unmet needs and to meet them. We started with St. Louis County at about $1.00 per capita and then it went to $1.50, all of it focused on target populations. This was an epidemiological approach rather than, "Let's just start a program in Cape Girardeau."

When I joined Western Missouri in February 1984, I was the first non-medical superintendent, for better or for worse. My focus was on internal programming and community relations. The publicity about the center was poor and many in Kansas City thought Western Missouri was not a good place. It had developed a reputation as a lockdown facility with a lot of security and had taken on the mantle of the state hospital. Because the other mental health centers were fresh and new at the time, it became the old, poorly maintained facility to serve people with serious illness. People were frightened of it. My goal was to make it more effective and more accessible.

I held the belief that this was a community agency that belonged to the people. We revitalized the center's advisory board and met with them on a regular basis. I moved security staff so we no longer looked like a police station. We redecorated the lobby. The thing that I would like to be remembered for is putting purple carpeting in the lobby. Most staff worried about carpets in patient areas. They said, "No, you've got to have tile in the lobby because the patients will urinate on the carpet and it will stink." They didn't, by the way. We tried to create an open environment. To me it was the most exciting job ever.

Tri-County was "reborn" in 1990. Beverly Sue Ryan, Harry Cleberg and Sandra Ferguson called me and said that the North Kansas City Hospital was getting out of the community mental health business. I was in private practice at the time and agreed to be a consultant to help create a new program. Beverly Sue, Sandra and I sat down and discussed the idea of a network model which relied on community providers as well as facility-based staff to deliver a service. They liked the idea. In June 1990, they got it incorporated and I served as the interim director. I was hired as the new CEO a few months later.

The network concept came from the Metropolitan Clinic of Counseling, which was a managed care organization that had set up shop in Kansas City. They had a small two-room office. They had two employees; they had a social worker and a secretary and they managed 25,000 covered lives for Blue Cross/Blue Shield. My first question when I met them was, "Where is your staff?" They said, "We don't have any staff; we put people in the network; we have providers who are in private practice. We assess the patients, we do the initial interview, and we figure out a treatment plan, put them in our network and monitor the results." I thought about how economical this concept was.

Once established, the new Tri-County needed to borrow $25,000 to meet payroll. We hired three people and promised to pay them later. Once we were incorporated, we were designated as the administrative agent for Clay, Platte and Ray counties. Our biggest opponent was Mike Benzen in central office who said, "You can't outsource all this money." My reply was, "Why not. The regional center does it all the time." Great Rivers was up and running, and I knew they contracted with private providers for much of their service. Great Rivers was started with less than 20 staff located at St. Louis County Hospital. The difference was that Great Rivers had POS contracts with their providers. DMH central office wouldn't allow POS contracts with my providers. All the contracts were with Tri-County, a single entity.

In the beginning, we were doing more network contracts: probably 20% with staff, 80% provider service. Over the years, we have reached a 50-50 ratio, although 60% of the revenue comes from the network. The hardest thing to protect has been the involvement of the network. Every time we hire new managers, their first impulse is to hire more staff. The critical part of the network is not the economics of it. The economics are great and we appreciate good financial results. The critical feature is our partnership with the community. We don't have competitors; we only have collaborators. The private practice base is infinite, insofar as they will always be willing to take one more patient.

RESPONSIBILITY FOR A SPECIFIED POPULATION: Defined service areas are still in place in Missouri. Very seldom do you see mental health centers crossing over into other people's territories. Even where service areas have combined, they still respect the integrity of the service areas and they still have local board ownership.

PREVENTION AND EARLY INTERVENTION: Prevention and early intervention efforts are certainly alive and well at Tri-County. We have 15 community teams with 15 different school districts and are probably spending upwards of $500,000 yearly on consultation or prevention services. For a while, DMH allowed us to bill 5% a year of our allocation for prevention. We get about $80,000 in prevention funds from the alcohol and drug division. The rest of that service is county supported.

Prevention makes a difference because it supports a model oriented to changing the community. Tri-County is more than a treatment entity to serve people who have serious mental illness. We are really here to "cure" the community of social ills, or at least address them. For example, through the Community 2000 program we promoted keg registration for beer distributors, so that law enforcement could track the kegs when minors were found with the booze. Local communities like Richmond have banned beer sales at their Mushroom Festival. These communities have been strengthened to organize around these social issues. It's not whether having beer is good or bad for the festival. The issue is for the leadership, the decision-makers, and the gatekeepers in those communities to be thinking about the public messages we give our youth. To get on board with the idea of, "This is a family affair and families can live without liquor, and we ought to promote good health," is the issue. Those interventions have been successful in changing community attitudes. Most importantly, it is the youth and community leadership working together on local issues. I think this process reduces stress and helps create better integrated, functional families.

If you want to look at prevention in a treatment context, what we do with some of the direct intervention programs like Family Preservation or Families First is instructive. Today we are not institutionalizing kids. Rarely do we have a youth more than ten days at a residential facility. We deliver in-home intervention, outpatient, medication management, community support and targeted case management together to keep the kids in their home. If part of our goal is to have people be self-sufficient, independent and autonomous in a least restrictive environment, then I think we are doing it.

Another thought I had while looking at the list of values we promote, is the close link we have with the public health model of intervention. It directs us to treat the whole community. We take an ecological approach or an epidemiological approach to an entire population. In addition to treating people who are sick, we focus on the entire population at-risk. That is clearly a public health sentiment. In general, you would call it a social change model. Even putting aside the idealism that we might eventually prevent schizophrenia or something like that, you can take a public health perspective on treatment. Fetal alcohol syndrome is an example. We know that if mothers who are about to give birth are drinking too much, it can affect the fetus, producing low birth weight and mental retardation. So you intervene with drug and alcohol programs, especially those that emphasize education and prevention.

TREATING PEOPLE IN THEIR HOME COMMUNITIES: Retaining people in the community is what we do. Inpatient care is vital when needed, but we admit fewer than 200 people a year. We provide a continuum of care for the target population. More than half of the 8,000 patients we see each year have a serious mental illness. Tri-County has 2,400 people in medication clinics; easily half of them have a serious mental illness, and the others have acute situational problems.

MULTIDISCIPLINARY TEAMS: We have multidisciplinary teams at all levels, as part of our community provider system and as part of our internal staffing. We also provide peer counseling with clients. We have several consumers trained as peer counselors who are on our payroll. DMH last year was trying to fund some of those positions and we have always had staff involved with the training. We have employed peer counselors for the last four years. It always made sense to me to involve some of our healthy consumers, the ones who are successful in their battles with mental illness. That is what our drop-in center is all about. We encourage people who are functional, so others can learn from them and see how it is done.

Multidisciplinary teams that include consumers is the ultimate expression of a team model. At Mid-MO, one of my first experiences involved ward government meetings with twenty patients in a circle and three or four staff asking people, "Do you think Mrs. Smith is ready to go home?" I thought, "What are you asking the patients for; what do they know?" But that is the methodology and the belief. We start with the assumption that consumers have strengths and they can express them. That consumers have something valuable to say about their treatment, is a vital starting point.

Medications, of course, help quiet symptoms so the problem-solving ability of people can be tapped. Thorazine was necessary before you could have a therapeutic community. The medications open the door for communication, but the community opens the door to independence.

LINKAGES WITH OTHER ORGANIZATIONS: Tri-County has 75 providers in our network. If collaboration was not a word when we got started, it is now. I don't know how we could be more collaborative or integrative or any combination of that. The agency is in the health department and in the hospitals; we are in the consumer's home and we have great staff and providers working as a team to serve our consumers.

CITIZEN PARTICIPATION: We have an active governing board. There are times when I think we could do more, but when I look at our community programs, I see we have nearly 300 volunteers who are involved with community drug education in the schools. These efforts provide strong threads in the social fabric of our communities.

Embedded in our social heritage is a belief about empowering everybody equally. Instead of going to an authoritarian medical model structure, everybody's voice becomes important. That was part of the civil rights movement, the social upheaval, the freedom marches and all the rest during the 1960s in this nation. That ethos is fundamental when you have a group of patients in a therapeutic community and you look to each of them to talk about their own destiny and talk about their own sense of whether they should be in the hospital. Everyone in the therapeutic community has a voice and that is why local control, local government, and local management in the global community are such important issues.

Instead of resting social controls in Jefferson City or Washington D.C., Tri-County has a real estate agent, an accountant, a teacher, a banker, etc. on our board. The first thing many of them will say when you try to get them on the board is, "I don't know anything about mental health," and I respond, "But you know about the community." So we start the conversation with that and it is empowering at a new level. We acknowledge and give credit to people who perhaps did not think of themselves as mental health experts. We emphasize, "Your voice is important."

For an example of community involvement that is working, I recall visiting in Monett with Frank Compton while he was creating a disaster response plan for tornadoes that devastated southwest Missouri. Frank had been there a long time, in a small community with limited resources. I imagined they were looking for instructions on what to do. Far from it. The truth is they were out there the day the tornado hit, and the following day they were working with the Red Cross supporting the first responders. They were linking with school personnel; they were in the community with their leaders. The agency was doing all the right stuff in the right sequence. They jumped on the crisis immediately and instinctively they got in the middle of it. They became part of the healing process for a community coping with disaster.

Community-based mental health services did not replace institutional care overnight. This was done gently over 40 years. Programs moved forward as the capability and desire of the community were increased to provide people with integrated supportive services – services located near family and friends. There is a woman in our community whose son had been in St. Joseph State Hospital for nearly ten years. With the introduction of new medications, she asked, "Can't you do something with my son and try him on Clozaril?" The state effort to move people into community support worked with this man once we treated him with Clozaril. Today he has a home. He lives part time with his family and part time on his own. His mother is delighted and she can't ever forget where her son was. This has to be a better place.

My background is nursing. I received a grant through NIMH to get my master's degree in psychiatric nursing at KU. Through that process, I was involved in a volunteer group to try to get mental health services to south Jackson County, Missouri. In 1968, we actually got services from a Western Missouri satellite clinic and Family and Children's Services. We got some money from the Kansas City Association for Mental Health, and a small 314 (d) grant from Dick Cravens at DMH helped us put in a phone. We opened in Sunday school classrooms at Unity Village. Professional staff saw clients there and volunteers staffed the office.

It was then necessary to raise $141,000 to match the federal CMHC construction grant. The match rate was 49%-51%. We raised the match, received a construction grant, and in the process business was growing in the offices at Unity Village, so we received an additional allocation from the state. We moved to what was the old Jackson County hospital, a former nursing home. The construction grant was awarded and then we went after a federal staffing grant. The staffing grant almost coincided with the completion of the building.

The community board of directors was organized in 1968 and I was the director of the organization. The board helped with fund raising and publicity. Initially, we were started by a ministerial alliance in Raytown. Then we pulled in school district representatives from Lee's Summit and Raytown, and then some of the prominent leaders in the area. Influential people in Lee's Summit arranged to have the land donated that we put our building on.

I totally believed in community mental health and involvement with the community. Actually, I never worked in a hospital setting. My background was always in the community. As a visiting nurse in Boston, I enjoyed relating with community people. The board of directors was very important to me. I spent a lot of time training the board and always believed that I never knew everything, but if I had the right people around me that had the knowledge, I would survive. I also felt that if you worked early in the community with some of these patients, either coming out of the hospital or before they went into the hospital, many of them could be cared for in the community. The front-door and the back-door roles were real important. I believed that mental health should be a part of total health care and it was very troubling to me that people did not understand mental illness. There was so much stigma attached to it. One of the themes we had when we ran our first county mill tax campaign was *No one is immune*. I liked that because immunity goes along with health and the fact is that no one exists who does not know someone who has a mental illness, either in their family or otherwise. At that time, nobody was admitting it.

When I was in nursing school in Boston, I toured one of the old state-run "insane asylums" at Danvers, Massachusetts. Our clinical experience was at the Boston Psychopathic Hospital. That was where my interest in mental health developed. We had a wonderful nursing instructor, Anne Hargraves. There were people in my neighborhood in Andover, Massachusetts, who were mentally ill, and we were not afraid of them. My mother was a nurse and she was very good with them, and so I felt comfortable with them.

There was a commitment to provide quality services and assure that the facilities we provided them within were not second class, and they were professional and that people were treated with dignity. The same standards that you would get in the health care field were really important.

When you're starting something from scratch without any money, you have to glue together a patchwork from many sources. So we went after United Way money through the Kansas City MHA, and then we got $26,666 in revenue-sharing dollars from Jackson County legislators to help build the building. Then we went after small grants to help with adding staff. We got some small grants from foundations. To build the building, we sold paper bricks in shopping centers. We also passed the mill tax levy.

I did not want to be the first director, even though I had brought the center to the point of writing the staffing grant and building the building. Ray Morgan was hired as the first director. He was there for two years, and then I was asked to assume the directorship to get the expansion grant in. I wrote the grant expanding from 5 to 12 services in 1974. That increased the services we provided, but the federal share was on a declining schedule. As we were getting near the end of our eighth year, we had no "big daddy" to assist us. It was at this time that we merged with a major health system. The merger provided enhanced cash flow, personnel benefits and technical assistance.

We were constantly looking for ways to get contracts and raise funds. The hardest part was always looking for money, always having your hand out. We got revenue-sharing dollars and contracts with Grandview, Lee's Summit and Raytown. We would get grants of $10,000 to $15,000 to help support our services. We had outreach offices in those cities so that there would be a visibility of services. When the CMHC Act was initiated, we were told that national health insurance was just a few years away. I believed it. What helped our centers in Jackson County were the mental health tax levy and the anti-drug sales tax. We were very involved in the county mental health and substance abuse taxes.

The whole time that the mental health centers were developing and strengthening, the state hospitals were downsizing and clients were coming back to the community. So the need was to use state dollars to help former state hospital clients who were coming back to the community; we went through a significant return of clients from St. Joseph State Hospital. Community placement got transferred to the mental health centers, so we had to work very hard at finding housing and at supervising care and medication clinics. The community-based services are such a critical part of the state services because the state hospitals have downsized and the mental health centers are the primary organizations that keep people in the community.

In Missouri, centers have tried to keep a balanced program, given the constraints of how you use state and Medicaid dollars. The idea was if we took general revenue, we could maximize those dollars with Medicaid and get more money. However, it really kind of sunk the ship in terms of using general revenue dollars for other than Medicaid. That was the push – to try to get more Medicaid dollars – but it caused a critical shift in services. We did not have a choice. It was going to be Medicaid, and we were told who could receive the services. There were a lot of people who were very ill and needed services, but if they were not Medicaid eligible, their services would not be funded. The whole focus was on the adults, although there were many kids with a serious emotional disturbance who might not have even had a diagnosis at that point. Funding does dictate services. If you want the dollars, you have to do what the money is designed for.

There are standards about what a CPR is supposed to be. Some of the standards are over and above some of the standards set by the Joint Commission. So even though centers are accredited by the Joint Commission, they have to get certified as a CPR program because DMH doesn't think that accreditation takes into account all the things that are important for community rehab. That philosophy is still in existence.

RESPONSIBILITY FOR A SPECIFIED POPULATION: If you're going to be a non-profit organization and get support from the community, having a designated community to relate to is important.

PREVENTION AND EARLY INTERVENTION: Prevention and early intervention have dwindled, unless you have separate sources of funding to do it. There is no consultation and education money anymore, unless you get some grants such as our mental health center does. We offer a sexual abuse prevention program called *What's the Secret?* that has been around for 15 years. We have to raise money for that and use volunteers to do it. There are more prevention dollars in drug and alcohol services.

We know so much more now about genetics and predispositions to mental illness, I'm not real comfortable with how you're going to prevent a mental illness that has a genetic origin.

TREATING PEOPLE IN THEIR HOME COMMUNITIES: Every mental health center that I know tries to keep people out of the hospital and find alternatives for them in the community. I think that's still a really high priority.

CONTINUUM OF CARE: Medication has become extraordinarily important for treatment; a psychiatrist has to be totally involved. The continuity of care coming out of the hospital and being able to get patients into medication clinics has been worked out. The assignment of a case manager to anyone who is in a medication clinic was a very, very wise move.

MULTIDISCIPLINARY TEAMS: Paraprofessionals are becoming increasingly more important because their salary is more manageable than Ph.D. level staff, but they need the supervision. You're going to find, as you do in the health care field today, that you will have physicians' assistants and nurse practitioners, that whole move toward less credentialed staff with supervision.

LINKAGES WITH OTHER ORGANIZATIONS: Linkages with other organizations have become more and more important because of the increased number of specialty agencies.

FISCAL AND PROGRAMMATIC ACCOUNTABILITY: I think that we in Missouri can take a lot of pride in the fact that we probably have one of the most accountable systems for managing public finances through the POS system, both at the state and the county levels. I feel that the Coalition of CMHCs, which formed a fiscal managers organization, has strengthened the fiscal accountability. We're getting public dollars and we must be accountable.

CITIZEN PARTICIPATION: Citizen participation was very important to me. I believe that the advocacy organizations such as NAMI have come into their own. I think the consumer groups are very important, as well.

Doug Hall is the CEO of Musselman and Hall Contractors of Kansas City, an asphalt, concrete and railroad construction and maintenance company founded by his grandfather in 1914. For the past 30 years, he has been active in services for persons with a mental disability at the state and local levels, including as a member of the board of directors of the Harry S Truman Children's Neurological Center near Lee's Summit, Missouri, a residential and day treatment facility for developmentally disabled children and adults.

From 1981 to 1985, Mr. Hall was Mayor of Raytown, Missouri. In 1973, he began his 30-year affiliation with the CMHC serving Raytown, then known as Community Mental Health Center-South, and recently renamed ReDiscover. He has served on the boards of directors of the center and its foundation and has been elected president of each. In 1984, Doug Hall's selfless contributions to improving care for persons with a mental disability and his outstanding business and political acumen were recognized by Governor Christopher Bond, who appointed him to the Missouri Mental Health Commission.

When I was president of the Raytown Jaycees in 1973, I met Shirley Fearon, who was selling paper bricks to help raise money to build the area's first CMHC building. Our Jaycee chapter got involved in a fund-raising program to make the federal match so they could fund the building. I guess she thought I had some potential because she asked me to be on the board of the Southeast Jackson County MHA in December 1973. I was on that board for a few months and they had an opening on the corporate board at the mental health center and so they asked me to join.

They were still in Unity Village at that time; they had not started construction on the new building yet. I observed the incredible energy of Shirley Fearon and the high level of dedication among the volunteers with whom she was involved. There was a complete lack of services out there in that area. It was pretty rural at the time. I lived out in Raytown, but it was in the country then; the city is growing around it right now.

I did not know very much about mental illness. It was only by mistake that I was on the center board because we had a daughter who was born with mental retardation in 1970, and I wanted to try to help her and learn about that system. I did not know at the time that there was a difference between mental retardation and mental illness. I looked at this as an opportunity to help my daughter and I ended up getting involved in the mental illness delivery system first. I knew nothing about mental illness at all, although I had been around some persons with alcoholism.

The first center board meeting was at Jackson County Public Hospital. That was ironic because I could see the hospital from my front yard when I was growing up; we always called it the county home. It was a place you did not want to go. It was terrible, a totally terrible place. At the time of my first meeting, they had just begun to renovate the facility and we had talked about the inpatient unit that ultimately opened there. We went over to look at where the unit was going to be; it was just a big ward that was completely empty. It was just a dream at that time.

The board was made up of banking people and civic leaders. The man who was the chairman was Ernie Doss, an insurance man in Raytown, as was Bill Reich, who was part of the group that started the Blue Ridge Bank and the Blue Ridge Mall. Mildred Raymond was the legal counsel. They were mostly people like that – bankers, insurance people. Of all the boards I have ever been on, and I have been on many boards, Shirley was the one person that knew the value of boards and knew how to cultivate the board so that they would be allies of hers. She did a great job.

The Raytown Jaycees got involved in the building campaign because at that time if you raised a quarter, the feds would match it with 75 cents. So the Jaycees raised about $1,500 to hire Holly

Carothers to be the receptionist and secretary. The Jaycees funded that first position.

Mildred Raymond thought that we needed to start a foundation so we could do fund raising and keep the contributions separate in the foundation and make them properly tax deductible. We were meeting one day in 1980 or so, and Bev Nicks reached in her pocket and pulled out $5 and said, "Here. I will make the first contribution." That became the development arm of the mental health center and we would raise money and put the money in the foundation and it now has close to a million dollars in it from that $5. For many years when the mental health center would generate a profit, we would take some of the profit and put it into the foundation. There have been significant contributions, board campaigns and that sort of thing and the fund raisers along the way have gone in there. Actually, about half of the money that we have raised has gone into the foundation, and the other half was spent on operations and special projects.

When the federal grant ran out, some people thought it was a good thing. It kind of kept our eye on the ball; it also was our impetus to get the county levy passed. When we got that done, we thought that money would go to the mental health centers, but at the very first meeting of the funders, fifty people showed up and wanted some of the money. We did not realize that we had that kind of competition. Anybody that ever administered any kind of services was standing there with their hand out. Many of them had very good political connections. That was an immediate battle that we did not expect to fight, but we fought it and the organization has been very well-funded with that group.

We used to go around to the cities and beg for money and actually would get some from time to time. The county gave us money a few times before the levy was passed. Raytown would give us a little; Grandview gave us some. So that was part of the fund-raising effort and you had to do that if you were going to stay in business.

151

Trying to stay on top of the inflation curve and trying to extend the services are why we ended up getting into the marriage with Research. Shirley thought that if this mental health center was ever going to be a viable professional organization, it needed to step beyond the church basement concept and find an ally that thought there was a value to community mental health. She called me one day and asked if I would meet with her and Dick Brown over at Research Hospital about joining forces. We all met and talked about the program. Research was looking to be more global at that time because it had just been a hospital organization and they thought they needed to be more integrated than they were.

They wanted a system and they saw some benefit to having the mental health center there. They saw some value in having their name on the mental health center and being able to show the community that they were supporting not-for-profit organizations. I don't think they quite realized the financial commitment they were going to make at the time. So they said they would do it, and the mental health center merged with Research and immediately took all of the employees into their benefits system and they became full-fledged employees of the organization, which was a huge improvement for all of the staff. When times got rough, they bailed us out. They really kept it hands-off. They let the board run the place. They put money into it and they would always brag about the mental health center and what a wonderful organization it was, but they had little input into what we were doing.

When Shirley left, Alan Flory came in. Shirley built it as a clinical program, but Alan built it as a business. He is one of the best I have ever seen.

They sold the entire Research system to HCA, except for the four not-for-profits. They have left behind a foundation that is operating the four not-for-profits, and they have given them orders to make a plan to separate themselves – to become independent.

Comprehensive Mental Health Services started in 1969 as an outreach office out of Western Missouri Mental Health Center. A nurse named Lorraine Nelson, who was an original employee of the Western Missouri outreach office, still works for us part time. We received a staffing grant in July 1974. Shortly after that, we got a construction grant that allowed us to buy our building in the Englewood area of Independence. The local hospital, which at that time was called the Independence Sanitarium and Hospital, provided the space for the mental health center and we had our inpatient unit there. The grants were both made to the Northeastern Jackson County Community Mental Health Center; in 1981, we changed our name to Comprehensive Mental Health Services.

When I came in October 1978, the center was really known for two basic services. We had the inpatient unit; other than Western Missouri, at that time there was not very much in the way of inpatient psychiatric services in this area. We also had a very strong outpatient program. All that we had for persons with a serious mental illness at that time were day treatment and case

153

management services. We did not have any residential group homes or anything like that. As a matter of fact, our group home was the first residential group home to open in Missouri. What we pretty much offered back in 1978 was a little less than a $1 million program. When Jim McKee left in 1982, I ended up becoming the director.

It has changed quite dramatically since then. We are not looked upon as the inpatient resource in the area because we no longer operate an inpatient unit ourselves. Much more, we are looked upon as a full-service organization with a strong emphasis in the schools. We have a school services department, whose staff work in about six different school districts in our area. We provide a wide range of services and at one time in our history, we operated an alternative school. Now we provide the mental health and substance abuse support services to the Northeast Jackson County alternative school.

We are also well-known for our crisis intervention, a reputation that predates ACI, the DMH crisis access system, especially our responses to natural disasters and manmade disasters, like the Hyatt Regency collapse. At that time, Richard Gist, our head of consultation and education, coordinated much of the early intervention work. We had a general philosophy about responding to disasters. One of the things that I brought to Comprehensive when I came was that, as a CMHC, we have to be concerned not just with the individual clients that need the services, but also with the mental health of the whole community. At that time we were reaching out to all the different fire departments and police departments and talking about how we could do critical stress debriefing and all of those kinds of things. When the Hyatt Regency collapsed, Richard and I said, "OK, we are going to get help down there." It was not in our service area but it was in our community. We became known for those kinds of things.

Later on, there was an incident at Planned Parenthood in Independence and we responded immediately with the workers and helped them recover from that crisis. We had a number of bank robberies and we ended up responding immediately to help the banks and help their employees recover. Several young children out here in the community who were ice-skating fell through the ice and died. We coordinated meetings, not only with the families and the schools, but also with the community, to deal with the grief. Then there was the case where the little boy got dragged behind a car a few years ago. It was a horrendous thing here in Independence and we had a whole series of community activities so people could deal with that and grieve about that. Responding to those kinds of disasters became sort of a trademark of Comprehensive.

Later on we were looking at the needs of people with a serious mental illness and we ended up going for a HUD Grant for Turning Point Group Home, which was really the first community-based psychiatric group home in Missouri.

We have branched out more into the substance abuse area which we were not heavily into. There was a stand-alone organization in Kansas City called Renaissance West that began at about the same time as Comprehensive which had been the primary provider of those services in the African-American community for Kansas City. Some years ago they reached out to us for consultation. After a lot of discussion, we decided to look at whether our two organizations should merge, and eventually Comprehensive took that service over. It was about thirty days from going out of business. Cliff Sargeon was chairman of the board at the time.

I am out here in eastern Jackson County in Independence, Missouri, and they are inner Kansas City. Some people would say the two organizations were geographically – but more so culturally and spiritually – removed, and yet this board was convinced that they should come to the assistance of this inner-city organization. For our board, this was really quite a big thing to think about. It is one thing to maybe come to the assistance of an organization of eastern Jackson County that is hurting. It's another thing to come to the assistance of an organization that is located in the inner city, but we did. It is working out very well, although we did have three tough years. We poured a lot of our assets and resources into the organization. I initially misjudged the amount of resources and

155

time and effort it would take to turn the situation around. Thankfully, the board did not throw me out the door on my butt. They hung in there with me, and today it is a strong, viable force within the community. It is now a department of Comprehensive Mental Health Services. I think it speaks volumes for the center and really volumes for the board of directors that ultimately came to the decision that it was a worthwhile endeavor to save this resource rather than see it go away.

The western region of DMH is very unique from a number of points of view. You have four mental health centers in Jackson County; we are unique with that. There are no lines on the street saying which service area you are in. In the beginning there was a lot of rivalry – rivalry for funding, rivalry for programming, rivalry on all kinds of levels among the mental health centers in this region. Over the years that changed and I think that is really a testament to the centers in this area. They started coming together more. As time went by, we adopted the philosophy that in order to improve the entire mental health system, everyone had to improve; you could not do it at the expense of each other. To fight when there were scarce resources to serve people was just not very wise.

The mental health levy helped a great deal. That was a vehicle to bring people together. We all had to come together to try to get this tax passed. In 1980 or so we went for a mental health levy tax and did not make it; it failed only by a little bit. Then we went back for the levy tax a couple of years later and we got it passed. It was a $3 million levy tax, and there was still a lot of competition then. The mental health centers and residential treatment centers came together to help push the tax. Then we really needed to go back to the taxpayers because it was not bringing in enough money. So we had another levy campaign spearheaded by the mental health centers and the children's residential treatment centers, and this time we decided to bring in a number of other organizations that had not really been recipients of the tax money but who needed help. We presented this to the public as a safety net issue that was going to help not one organization but all of these organizations working together cooperatively to provide a coordinated system of mental health care. We got that tax passed.

Then the mental health levy board put together a committee that had to hammer out the details of how funding should go, what the structure of the system should be, and everything else. That plan is still followed to this day.

I think that helped set a philosophy that allowed us to address the issue of CommCare, which was the big defining issue for our region. It was our response to managed care and our response to the state's MC+ program effort. We started thinking about CommCare before there was MC+. We were at Shirley Fearon's office one day talking about managed care coming in and where we were going to end up under managed care. I said that we needed to market directly to insurance companies. We each assigned a staff member – I assigned Ray Morgan, Shirley assigned Mel Fetter, and each of us assigned somebody to just put together a marketing strategy. The insurance companies did not want to deal with us one at a time. That was in 1994. We had to adopt some of the trappings of the private sector to compete successfully.

We first were working and meeting together to develop some marketing strategies and approaches; then we put up some money to capitalize that. We each put up $2,500. That was our starting war chest. We wanted to be able to make application to MC+ but could not because Missouri wrote the rules that the only people who could apply to MC+ were bona fide healthcare systems or the insurance industry, and we were neither of those entities. We had to market ourselves to whomever was going to get the awards. In Jackson County there were four awards granted. We went to each one of the awardees and marketed ourselves as the behavioral health part. In the beginning, we had a contract with each one of them; we had some contractual arrangements with all of them in different ways, and rates varied from program to program. They were somewhat comparable to what we were getting from the state for POS. We bought an interest in a regional managed care company in four states here. CommCare is one of the greatest things we ever did; it is what really sets us apart. It is mental health centers being managed care entities, with a heart. We are in it to do good things and to try to make money.

RESPONSIBILITY FOR A SPECIFIED POPULATION: This is still operational, although it is not totally strictly adhered to, because in being responsible for an area, we find that we cannot do it by ourselves. So, we end up sharing our resources with other service agencies that are responsible for an area.

PREVENTION AND EARLY INTERVENTION: Still very much in vogue but very difficult to carry out because of fiscal constraints. There is some limited availability of our POS funds for those kinds of activities. Our county dollars also help pay for some of those activities, largely through the COMBAT drug and alcohol funding, which has a prevention piece built into its structure.

TREATING PEOPLE IN THEIR HOME COMMUNITIES: Absolutely. This is a high priority; that is why we are more into the group home business, more into apartments and more into assisted living and those kinds of things.

CONTINUUM OF CARE: That is the major principle that defines us – service delivery that is a full-service continuum of care. Traditional outpatient has morphed a lot, with managed care influences. Outpatient therapy relies more on psychoeducational approaches. It is still a service that we provide.

Cultural competence has been one of the major emphases in change within our service delivery system from the beginning. Early on, we were primarily talking about just giving services to the community – giving psychotherapy, doing day treatment, whatever. It was a cookie-cutter approach. A person walked in and if you had a particular treatment philosophy that you practiced, then you practiced it when they came in the door. Then they got it and if they did not get better, then shame on them. Over the years we recognized that as far as the effectiveness of our treatment is concerned, it doesn't just depend on the treatment techniques that we have, in terms of who responds to what; rather, the best treatment for people depends on cultural backgrounds, ethnicity, religious issues and other things.

We started doing outcome studies and learned that certain people were not getting better in our systems, particularly people of color, be that Asian, Latino, American Indian or African-American. The majority culture was getting much better and we wondered if it was because of differential treatment. We learned that it was because our treatments were not tailored to our clients. The access was really distorted: the majority culture was accessing our services at a much higher rate, even though when we looked at the prevalence of mental illness, we knew there was lots of need in the non-majority communities and they were not accessing us because the treatments that we were doing were not relevant. We had so many institutional biases.

MULTIDISCIPLINARY TEAMS: The paraprofessionals have grown by leaps and bounds with all the emphasis on case management, personal care attendants, etc. In some instances we do use peer counselors for recovery. By paraprofessionals we are defining anybody who does not have an advanced degree. That really covers the large number of case managers who are working with persons with a serious mental illness in particular and a large number of mental health techs that we use in all of our operations.

LINKAGES WITH OTHER ORGANIZATIONS: This is crucial for our being able to survive and that is the whole thing behind our CommCare, the whole thing behind our levy taxes and substance abuse taxes. But now, it is much more collegial in how we run as a mental health community and how community mental health centers go forth to better serve our clients.

FISCAL AND PROGRAMMATIC ACCOUNTABILITY: That is the key to survival in tight financial times. We have much better systems and we are under the gun so much more. We get our funding from multiple sources. I have always said it takes about a hundred funding sources to make a mental health center functional. Every one of those funding sources, if they give you a dime or a million dollars, wants strict accountability. They all audit you multiple times a year, so we spend more time accounting for the money than we do acquiring it and using it. Outcome studies and fiscal reviews make sure that this money only goes for the services it is supposed to and only to the people who are authorized to get them.

CITIZEN PARTICIPATION: We are still run by community boards of directors and various advisory boards. The community still dictates what kind of services it wants.

MISSOURI FIRST-PERSON INTERVIEW WITH:
TODD D. SCHAIBLE, PH.D.

Dr. Todd Schaible has served as a chief executive officer in the mental health field for nearly 30 years, as president/CEO of Burrell Behavioral Health since its inception over 26 years ago. Under his leadership, Burrell has received local, state and national recognition for its innovation, broad continuum of care, initiatives in health/ behavioral health integration and children's services, and for its community service. Burrell is the only organization to have received three National Excellence Awards from the National Council for Community Behavioral Healthcare, including the Lifetime Achievement Award presented to Dr. Schaible. He began his career as a clinical psychologist and director of children's services. His early frustration at the lack of available services for children began an administrator's career and a reputation for innovation and entrepreneurship.

In 1976, Judge Don Burrell, John Sweeney, Dave Woodruff and several other Springfieldians enlisted the services of Dr. Stanley Peterson, a local physician active in community development, to write a CMHC grant application. Dick Cravens had alerted the judge that there would be some funds available in that year's federal CMHC allocations and, if they would get a grant application in, they would likely be funded. They did and it was. In late 1976, I was recruited to come to Springfield to take on the start-up of the then d.e. Burrell Community Mental Health Center. On January 3, 1977, I began work in what has remained my position for over 26 years.

Burrell began clinical operations in May 1977 and over the following year put in place the typical continuum of services dictated by the federal operations grant. But, I believe we had some distinct advantages in our start-up. We were coming on line more than a decade after the CMHC movement had started and we could draw from a wealth of other CMHC experiences. We had no preexisting operational base and therefore didn't have the burden of various legacy systems and operational cultures; we didn't have the push-back to do things a certain way because they had always been done that way. As it turned out, with the onset of the block grants in the early 1980s, we had the advantage of only receiving three years of the anticipated eight years of operation grants. I say advantage because eight years of grant dependency could have created an operational culture incompatible with the systems of accountability required by the real world of multiple customers and multiple sources of revenue. We were weaned early. As for the onset of block grants, we were further blessed by a state mental health department that had instituted a fee-for-service system of payment under the block grant program. I will always be grateful that in early debates, "payment for services provided" prevailed over "payment for a promise to provide services" to DMH.

Another distinct advantage for Burrell's development (although at times it was also a distinct disadvantage) was the lack of a state hospital conveniently available to our service area. Not having a state hospital nearby meant that there was no pressure valve that could be easily tripped, allowing a person to be admitted to the hospital in response to a problem that was best addressed by a lesser response. There was a greater impetus for Burrell to develop that lesser response. Of necessity, Burrell established systems of care in our community capable of effectively responding to higher levels of acuity than we would have if we had had ready access to a state hospital. Fairly early in our history we implemented programs such as group homes, semi-independent apartments, a stabilization and clinical respite facility, professional parent homes, home-based services, etc. I think that it was the absence of a quick and easy response for the more acute clients that gave us a clearer view of why clients had progressed to their level of acuity; how we had failed them; how we could, as our mission states, "meet mental health needs where and when they occur and before they become more serious."

This process of evolving from failure and necessity was further accelerated in the late 1980s and early 1990s with the closure of

Nevada State Hospital which, while distant from our service area, had taken some of the most acute patients from our area. During the same period, the inpatient children's units serving our area were closed at Mid-MO and Fulton State Hospital. As I recall, with the closure of the children's units, we received a third of the state's associated cost savings with which we now serve three times as many kids as a result of being able to respond with less intense and less restrictive levels of care. Our system of care for that population continues to evolve as we learn from our failures and attempt to plug the holes in the continuum in the context of limited and often inflexible reimbursement systems.

Engraved on a granite wall at the entrance of Burrell's central office is this phrase: "In all things there is opportunity." This is a message both for the people whom we serve as they confront their personal challenges and for ourselves as we confront our professional challenges as well. Early in Burrell's existence, we repeatedly encountered roadblocks in locating adequate offices: zoning and NIMBY (not in my back yard) obstacles in the north Springfield area and good-old-boy politics in the downtown area. Eventually, in an effort to avoid unwilling neighbors, we bought a 90-acre farm on the south edge of the city at the price of 12 cents a square foot, financed by a private estate, absent willing bank financing. We placed extensive restrictions on the property to insure its long-term value and integrity. Today, that "no neighbors" area is known as the Medical Mile, and the only remaining 1.5 acre parcel adjacent to Burrell Park would sell for more than what Burrell paid for all 90 acres. The proceeds from the sale of our excess property financed our central offices as well as other elements of our expansion. It is meaningful, and I believe instructive, that while in the beginning we weren't able to locate next to a hospital or medical and other professional office, in the end, hospitals and medical and professional offices were built next to a mental health center.

In 1994, Burrell took the important step of affiliating with Cox Health Systems (now CoxHealth). If we were going to meet mental heath needs where and when they occurred and before they became more serious, we certainly needed to integrate with health care. Cox made a major commitment to the development of mental health services and we became the health system's exclusive provider of behavioral health services. Over time, the health system has increasingly become the context of mental health service delivery. Not only has the hospital grown its inpatient psychiatry programs in response to community need, behavioral health services have been integrated into a number of specialty areas such as cardiology, endocrinology, oncology, physical and neuro rehab, etc. We also have placed mental health specialists in various outpatient medical clinics.

Our experience in all of these instances has validated our earlier real estate lesson. Create value experienced by those with whom you wish to deal, by those who will, in part, control your success. In placing mental health specialists in a medical clinic, we have failed when we did not go beyond simply co-habitating an office area. In those instances, we failed, not because we didn't provide valuable mental health services to our clients, per se; but rather because we didn't provide value to the larger context of the clinic. We have succeeded in our integration efforts when we have brought value to the doctors, the nurses, the receptionists, and yes, the accountants. It is in these contexts where mental health services over time are increasingly woven into the day-to-day functioning of the clinic through screening tools, bi-directional consults, system changes, changes in the report formats to make them more meaningful, etc. Burrell has repeatedly found this to be true in other co-location efforts with community entities such as health departments, schools, Division of Family Services, juvenile justice, Jordan Valley (a community health center), and others.

As we have pursued diversification and a broader continuum of services, there has been a dangerous counter-trend toward narrowing the range of services supported by DMH funding. I am referring to the broader and broader use of the Medicaid waiver mechanism to bring federal dollars into mental health services. While much good is done with these resources, there is a narrowing of the population and levels of acuity once served with DMH dollars, as those funds are increasingly used for Medicaid match. In the not-so-distant past, if you had a mental illness and needed services, you either waited until your need was serious enough to warrant hospitalization or you were hospitalized and received more services and utilized more resources than your condition required. As states, in pursuit of federal dollars, have narrowed their range of supported service, this too little, too much, too late, too early dilemma may be re-emerging. On the other hand, it is increasingly up to CMHCs to diversify their funding as a means of diversifying services, and it is that which may be the silver lining of this danger.

One of the blessings for CMHCs in Missouri was their formal designation as administrative agents of DMH, and I still believe that. As administrative agents, we were able to focus our energies on providing services, not on fighting for the right to provide services. But, in so doing and by virtue of our designation, we also largely defined who we were and what we did by what services DMH bought. As a result, maybe we haven't become as accomplished as we could have in "marketing" our services to a more diverse range of payers. Should we fail at that effort now, we may well abandon the notion of a network of "comprehensive" community mental health centers to a system of independent, and often uncoordinated, clinical entrepreneurs, each offering a narrow piece of the continuum with clients receiving the service being sold behind the door they happen to open.

Another very large plus for the long-term stability of Missouri's community mental health system, is the Missouri Coalition of Community Mental Health Centers. With the constancy of Kathy Carter's leadership over the past 25 years, a vehicle has reliably operated to insure a modicum of order: order in advocacy, in conflict resolution, in prioritization, in DMH and legislative relations. And a focus on *mission* rather than on individual member advocacy has persisted. In many ways, the Coalition has been the glue in the long-term and remarkable partnership between DMH and its community-based administrative agents, the CMHCs of Missouri.

RESPONSIBILITY FOR A SPECIFIED POPULATION: Whereas we once had exclusive responsibilities for a defined geographic service area, and we still do by virtue of our administrative agent role, we also have multiple populations that we are responsible for as a result of our relationships with various other payer sources or institutions. For us, the best example may be our exclusive provider status with Cox and its various insurance products, managed care contracts, etc., in the context of Cox's service area, which is much larger than our administrative agent service area. Over time, these types of relationships for CMHCs will likely be many and varied. They will strengthen or weaken our statewide Coalition and our "system" of care depending upon how we collectively and individually manage the potential conflicts and opportunities.

PREVENTION AND EARLY INTERVENTION: Over the past year, Burrell has spent a lot of time evaluating ways and means to more meaningfully provide prevention services, particularly in the area of children, as we have planned our new Center for Child and Adolescent Development. On one hand, we do a good bit now. We are in ten health department Women and Infant Children (WIC) clinics providing education to young parents, we reach over 2,000 parents a year in our Children First education program, we provide school-based suicide prevention programs, we offer various Employee Assistance Program classes and much more. In our thinking about kids, we are increasingly biased toward the notion that when a child has been brought to us because of a "problem," we should view that as a marker for a kid, that we should steer these very kids into various skill development programs and focus on where there is to go instead of what they must stop doing.

CONTINUUM OF CARE: It is ironic that one of the most pressing needs in our community, like in others across the state, is that of inpatient psychiatry. Last year alone we had to transfer 487 patients from Cox emergency room to other psychiatric units throughout the state because no beds were available. While we have expanded inpatient psychiatry at Cox to 69 beds, we remain full pretty much all the time. Several factors are contributing to this problem: many hospitals have reduced their psychiatric beds; those in the MR/DD population who are in crisis are increasingly referred to general psychiatric units as are the alcohol and drug addicted in times of crisis. Interestingly, the large number of folks who have a serious and persistent mental illness are very infrequent users of our inpatient beds. One step I believe we need to take across the state is to make available case managers to those who enter private and public hospital psychiatric units. Make every effort to connect them to a system of care and to gain eligibility to Medicaid, which will in turn enhance their access to that care.

MULTIDISCIPLINARY TEAMS: As we, like other CMHCs, continue to evolve, *what we do, where we do it, who pays* for it, and *who we serve* will all continue to change, as will *who does it.* We continue to evaluate those changes with an open mind but with an eye always on that basic mission which has served us well all these years: meet mental health needs where and when they occur and before they become more serious; provide as much care as is needed but no more than is needed. I can give you a recent example of a shift in our thinking about who provides a service and its relevance to our underlying mission. The question had been raised as to how many hearing impaired people we serve. As it turned out, we serve very few and those had fairly serious conditions. In response, we have added a counselor who is trained in communicating with the hearing impaired (In the past you would have had to have a third person in the counseling sessions to facilitate communication.) and have begun a system-wide evaluation of the barriers to access by the hearing impaired. Nurse practitioners taking on a portion of the work previously done by psychiatrists, nutritionists working with certain of our client populations, and parent and child advocates becoming part of the intervention process are all shifts in service provision in various stages of implementation.

Co-locating our staff in other settings, both medical and social service, will do much toward mutual awareness of opportunities to intervene earlier in an evolving mental health need. As I said earlier, we have psychologists in clinics and in the emergency room. We will not consider our success in those settings solely by whether or not our staff meets the mental health needs of patients in those settings. Rather, over time, another important marker will be whether other professionals working in those settings with

167

increasing frequency meet the mental health needs of those they encounter. And, just as we pursue the co-location of our staff in these various settings, we too must explore the potential synergies of others such as primary care providers integrating into our various service locations. Toward this end, our new Center for Child and Adolescent Development now under construction includes a Community Partners Wing with six partner offices as well as conference and meeting rooms. And the facility will have the necessary provisions built into the structure to accommodate medical clinics.

CITIZEN PARTICIPATION: You asked about consumer participation. First, we are all potential consumers and a pretty high percentage of us are actual consumers. Since the vast majority of families in the United States will have a member receive mental health services at one time or another, most of us are consumers.

Second, all consumers aren't alike. All mental illnesses are not alike. All those in a given age group are not alike. All those in a given ethnic group are not alike. If we want to know about barriers to using or benefiting from our services, we certainly do not want to rely on a sample of one or two representatives of any presumed group. We have available to us research tools to properly answer the questions we should be asking. For example, we want to know why persons 60 and older are such infrequent users of service when we know that folks in that age group experience a myriad of very serious mental health problems. Perhaps we need a separate *Issues of Aging Clinic* or a *Memory Clinic* rather than expecting that population to use a mental health clinic. Knowing the wants and needs of those we serve is vitally important and we should answer the necessary questions by the use of legitimate research tools and techniques.

As we pursue further development of our continuum of care, new partners in the delivery of services and new sources of funding, and we face the challenges ahead, we do so with full belief in the inscription on the granite wall as you enter our building: "In all things there is opportunity for growth.....value what you are and what you can become."

168

Karl Wilson, Ph.D. is the CEO of Crider Center for Mental Health, a position he has held for over 24 years. He received his doctorate in clinical psychology from the University of Florida, with emphasis in community psychology, and began his professional career in 1976, teaching at Washington University in St. Louis, where he still co-teaches a course in mental health policy. He has chaired the boards of a number of organizations, including the MHA of Greater St. Louis, Behavioral Health Response and the Missouri Coalition of Community Mental Health Centers. He currently serves on the boards of the Missouri Foundation for Health and several community human service organizations.

Crider Center for Mental Health primarily serves the Missouri counties of Lincoln, Warren, St. Charles and Franklin. These are fast-growing collar counties in the metropolitan St. Louis area. Our first name was the Mental Health Council of Lincoln, Warren and St. Charles Counties. It evolved from three state-run traveling clinics from Malcolm Bliss Mental Health Center in St. Louis. They would come out to St. Charles one day a week for kids and families and two days a week for adults. They also would go out to a church in Troy and the health department office in Warrenton. Traveling clinics from St. Louis State Hospital were the predecessors of the Mental Health Council of Franklin County, which was a separately incorporated organization. It started in borrowed space in hospitals in Sullivan and Washington. The Mental Health Council of Lincoln, Warren and St. Charles Counties incorporated in 1978 and began services June 30, 1979. The board, which included Jane Crider, had received consultation from the Malcolm Bliss staff.

When I was in my psychology internship at Malcolm Bliss in 1974-1975, I went out to traveling clinics at Murphy Blair and

Yeatman Union Sarah in north St. Louis. These traveling clinics eventually became Hopewell Center. I also spent one day a week in St. Charles, riding out with Bonnie DiFranco, who was a social worker at Malcolm Bliss at the time.

In 1979, while an assistant professor in the psychology department of Washington University, I heard that the Mental Health Council of Lincoln, Warren and St. Charles Counties had started delivering services. This group started losing money from day one and was using up a $10,000 donation from Jane Crider pretty quickly. The rates the board had negotiated with DMH were about half of the norm for other centers in Missouri.

In mid-August the board appointed me executive director at 10% time. I promised to do whatever was necessary to get the job done (which was about five times that level). I would not come back to them for an increase until the center grew enough that the overhead could be justified. I quickly learned there were a number of things that could be tightened down to increase productivity and control costs, but the basic problem was rate structure. We heard that there was a new director of DMH, Dr. Paul Ahr, and we met him at a hotel in Columbia before he officially began his position. Helping us was probably the first thing he did as DMH director. We sat down with DMH staff and came up with new unit rates. Within a month, our finances started to turn around.

It was like a honeymoon for the next six months as we grew. The next year we got a $250,000 DMH contract. I took a part-time leave and cut back to half time at the university. At the end of that year, they told me I had to either come back full time or give up the tenure track. I did not spend ten seconds on that. I gave up the tenure track, and 22 years later I am still teaching a course a semester.

I immediately investigated the federal CMHC grant application process. The most problematic part was providing inpatient care. The role that DMH saw for us was to take care of people that were being discharged from institutions. They did not have as high a priority on diverting people from being admitted in the first place.

I think by that point one of the issues for the states was that many federally funded centers were beginning to be phased out of their grants and the states saw this as a fiscal time bomb. DMH thought it could fund aftercare centers, but only a limited number of comprehensive community mental health centers.

Our CMHC grant was approved in January 1981. When Ronald Reagan became president, things changed dramatically with these grants. Our CMHC grant had already been reduced from over $1 million to about $600,000. Then 25% was taken away from the remainder and converted into the new block grant to Missouri. So I went to DMH to find our money, which was now about $450,000. DMH had agreed to continue to pass through the funding to the centers that had been funded when this conversion occurred. We ended up with about $250,000. Obviously, we were not going to do all of the things we would have under the federal grant and the state certainly had no requirements to start all these federally required programs. We converted most of it to expansion of our outpatient care but we held back on enough to begin prevention programs in the schools and an early intervention program for beginning school children. We called the program Pinocchio and it was a replication of Emory Cowen's very successful program in Rochester, New York. By this time, DMH was reorganizing new service areas from the old catchment areas and we absorbed the staff of the Mental Health Council of Franklin County and renamed ourselves Four County Mental Health Services.

Within our area there were two programs that had originated out of St. Louis State Hospital and had been partial replications of the 500-year-old foster community program in Gheel, Belgium. They were called Troy Foster Community and New Haven Foster Community. The whole point of it was to get a town to have ownership of a program that would help individuals coming out of institutions who no longer had a home community. St. Louis State Hospital provided training both to the soon-to-be-discharged patients and community volunteers with whom they would be matched. Ultimately, St. Louis State Hospital asked us to take over both programs. These evolved into our community support programs and rehabilitation centers, including Headway in St. Charles and Harmony in Washington. We followed the lead of Independence Center in adopting the Fountain House model for these clubhouses.

At the beginning, we needed to provide a psychiatric group home. We looked for an existing building. We ended up buying an empty boarding home for seniors that had gone out of business. Eventually, we came to the conclusion that the approach of moving people along a continuum of residential placements did not work well. When people adjust to a residential program, it becomes their home. Eventually, people adjust and stabilize so we tell them, "Congratulations; you are going to graduate." In essence, we were punishing them for getting better. So, we decided to bypass the group home wherever we could, placing people directly in the community and giving them a lot more support. We have more of a continuum now, but our ideas have changed in terms of providing support for individuals. What we are trying to do is reinforce the situations that they are in or help them find a permanent situation for themselves, to become a part of their community and develop their own networks. We give whatever support is needed. We still have the group home, but it is used for individuals who repeatedly fail in the community and would otherwise remain in the few long-term state beds. It's a slow process, but we have been successful in helping members find jobs and eventually get their own apartments.

The thing that I regret the most is that in the original federal grant application we were going to be able to do a lot more in terms of short-term counseling for people in the community. We would have helped with problems in everyday life and also in mental illnesses that were transitory. We have had to narrow our focus given state funding priorities.

RESPONSIBILITY FOR A SPECIFIED POPULATION: As a community mental health director, I take responsibility for the overall mental health of the people who live in our area. We have direct responsibility for a compressed range of services due to our insufficient pool of resources. We quantify the mental health needs of each target population. We then catalogue resources addressing these needs and we subtract that from the overall needs. What is left we calculate as being our community's unmet mental health needs. Some of these needs have not been manifested in demand because people don't translate all of their problems as being mental health problems, even when they are. When we look at the unmet needs, which are many times what we can do with the resources we have, tough rationing decisions have to be made. This is the role of the community board. We have to stop thinking in terms of being providers of a set package of services. We need to think in terms of what the needs are out there and then decide what the highest priority is. We then search for and develop the most effective and efficient tools to produce the best outcomes for the target population.

To carry out the mission of a community mental health center, it is necessary to have a local resource base. State and federal funding, Medicaid and Medicare, etc., are all important, but they are narrowly targeted and there will inevitably be holes in the service delivery system. We are disappointed that we have not been able to pass a local tax initiative to create local funds to fill gaps. Some centers have that and we do not as yet. We have built up United Way forms of charitable support, but this is not enough to cover the biggest gaps. We have used these charitable funds for prevention and early intervention, but have limited capacity to help "the working poor" who are not seriously mentally ill.

We still have a huge variation in Missouri between service areas in per capita funding. We now have over 480,000 people in our four-county area and had only 250,000 people twenty years ago. The problem is that although we have gotten new funding, our target keeps shifting because of our continuous growth.

PREVENTION AND EARLY INTERVENTION: There is a lot of talk about prevention, but few resources are committed to it. Some of the problem is that several decades ago there were few effective prevention tools. Now there are a number of evidence-based programs. Getting sustained funding for population-based mental health promotion and early intervention is a huge challenge.

For our mental health promotion strategy, we sought to have a population-based impact. We chose school-age children because access is a lot easier. We developed a program for preadolescents called *Changes and Choices*, a life skills program that gets built into the school curriculum. We just come in and take over a class. Over 60% of all sixth graders in our service area go through this course each year.

In 1995, the community mental health centers in metropolitan St. Louis decided to combine our resources to start a regional crisis-access system. Besides Crider Center, this included Hopewell, COMTREA, Great Rivers and St. Louis Mental Health Center. (The latter two became BJC BH.) The result was BHR, which receives over 11,000 calls a month from the region and provides mobile outreach in emergencies.

Crider Center for Mental Health has been a part of more federal disaster counseling grants than any other community mental health center in the country. Our first was in 1982, and included working with families relocated because of dioxin from Times Beach. Our largest was working with 10,000 families who were displaced by the great flood of 1993. Having the service area that includes the confluence of the two greatest rivers in the country has presented us with this challenge, and each time we have responded more comprehensively, we have developed a model for helping individuals, families and communities rebuild following disasters. The model has been used in disasters around the country. Again, it is a partnership model. In 1993, we had nine organizations in a single location collaborating on bringing comprehensive recovery services to survivors.

CONTINUUM OF CARE: At the beginning, our long-term plan was that we were going to develop a continuum of care. We conceptualized the continuum as a pyramid. At the base, horizontally, were mental health promotion and early intervention; right above that on the next layer was crisis intervention. On a third layer, we would have counseling, psychiatry and other outpatient services; the layers above that became much more complex over time. We found that rather than those layers being horizontal, they worked better if we had them side-by-side. These include community support, rehabilitation, employment supports, housing, etc. At the top, in the smallest space, is inpatient care. Later on, I realized that that continuum does not make any sense in terms of talking about the whole population; you have to have a continuum, a pyramid, for each target population. We had to think in terms of what are we doing about kids? What are we doing about adults? What are we doing about the elderly?

For the continuum of care to become a system of care, we have to then look at what degree does it partner up with the natural environment in order to multiply the impact of each one of these tools. Do we have relationships with natural caregivers where, as soon as people begin to break down, we are mobilized with our tools? Are we partnering with the natural caregivers in their own environment and offering consultative services to them? Over time we have learned ways of using our funding and other scarce resources to achieve better outcomes.

We have three target populations: for adults challenged with serious mental illness, we do whatever it takes in order to help the individual thrive in the community; for children who are challenged with serious emotional disturbance and their families, we help the child stay at home, progress at school and stay out of trouble. For the general public, we provide mental health promotion and early intervention programs at developmental change points. We try to assess what skills individuals need in order to thrive during the next stage of their lives; we find a gatekeeper who can give access to that general population and we then work on life skill development with that group. We have very short-term crisis-oriented counseling services. We are really doing triage and we are picking up those individuals who have the highest needs for more intensive intervention. Counseling is on a limited basis, provided by others, and so it ends up being a real luxury for us to provide. We would love to provide it. When we are successful in passing a local tax for mental health, there will be a lot more local pressure to deal with general public issues, including access to counseling services.

TREATING PEOPLE IN THEIR HOME COMMUNITIES: What works the best, what gives the best outcomes, is to take the services directly to our target populations (e.g., home- and school-based interventions). The state has told us to take care of people with the most serious problems first. So what we do is not wait until people come out of hospitals to offer services. We go out and find them. We are finding lots of them. We are finding them in the juvenile justice system that, up to six years ago, we had never touched before. We are finding adults who have a variety of mental health problems, so a crisis access system was needed. We need to provide short-term intensive interventions, and then we need a range of supports and services in order to help people to adapt in the community. We wrap those services around the client and we want to tailor the services to that individual and not do any more than we need to do.

We have been successful at convincing the schools to let us work with kids in their own classrooms. We call it school-based mental health consultation, while the schools call it education support counseling. We'll work either as crisis interveners or add mental health services on top of alternative school programs. This is a very cost-effective intervention, comparable to day treatment, and results in good outcomes. The cost of these services is split among the school, charitable funding (e.g. fund raising), United Way and billed services to DMH.

There are some major cultural differences between community mental health centers and schools. The original values of community mental health are wonderful, but these values don't automatically translate into being effective in these settings. Developing the tools that are consistent with those values took some time around the country. Finding and adapting these tools and putting them together into a coherent package continue to be our major challenge.

A major issue we face in services to children is "silos" or dissipation of responsibility and resources among a number of "authorities." The child welfare, education and juvenile justice systems had more resources, at one point, for children's mental health than the state mental health system in Missouri. This is changing, but these silos need to be broken down and services integrated in a system of care. We are proud to have brought to St. Charles County in 1997 the first federal grant to develop a local system of care in Missouri.

MULTIDISCIPLINARY TEAMS: The use of multidisciplinary teams has increased. We are committed to continually work on improving quality and improving the effectiveness and efficiency of our interventions. Part of that is a matter of testing the limits of what can be done with paraprofessionals. For example, in our children's program, the first person to walk in the home is the parent partner, rather than the master's-level care coordinator. The parent partner does a strengths-based assessment of the family and really makes an attachment, becoming an advocate for the family. The parent partners are usually women who have raised kids who have had a serious emotional disturbance, and so they have been there and done that. They are key components of our system. We need to develop a career track for them with our organization. We try to pay them well, but we lose many of them because the state's rates are so low for this service and for our family assistants.

LINKAGES WITH OTHER ORGANIZATIONS: It became apparent to us over time that in order for us to make a difference, we had to work through organizations that had better access to our target populations. Our effectiveness depended on how close we could get within natural settings, particularly with kids. We worked on getting partnerships with the 23 school districts in our area. This is a major challenge given the variation in size and complexity of the districts.

CITIZEN PARTICIPATION: The key to our survival as a community mental health center is developing strong stakeholder groups and strong partnerships. We do a lot to identify and work with stakeholder groups, partnering with them and creating ways of being accountable to them. In every county we have a system of care board where we sit down once a month and they tell us what is working and what is not working and we do planning with them. We continue to build our accountability to the community.

177

We have three judges on our board, three former legislators, school administrators, a former presiding county commissioner, business people, NAMI members, a Division of Family Services director, consumers and family members. We know our legislators and our stakeholders know our community.

Crider Center for Mental Health is in its 25th year of operations. We take seriously our role as the community mental health center for Lincoln, Warren, Franklin and St. Charles counties. We have a great board of directors, great management team, competent and dedicated staff, and terrific partners. We are building ourselves to last and to continuously improve in meeting our mission.

5 PARTNERING WITH THE STATE (1980-2003)

In September 1979, Paul R. Ahr, Ph.D., M.P.A., replaced interim DMH director, Beverley Wilson, M.D. Earlier that year, C. Duane Hensley, Ph.D., had resigned after two years as director. Within weeks of Ahr's arrival in Missouri, State Representatives Wayne Goode and Steve Vossmeyer met with him to discuss their interest in updating the bulk of Missouri's mental health statutes, which had not been revised in the state's major reorganization legislation five years earlier. The Mental Health Commission, Representatives Goode and Vossmeyer, and Ahr decided to move ahead with an overhaul of these statutes in the 1980 General Assembly. DMH's efforts were coordinated by Reginald Turnbull, chief counsel for the department on assignment from the Attorney General's office, who helped draft the Omnibus Mental Health Bill (H.B. 1724). As passed, this bill revised 90 sections of the mental health statutes and added 92 new sections. Of special interest to persons concerned about the ongoing contributions of the state's CMHCs were new sections:

1. Requiring DMH to identify in each geographic area of the state community-based services to serve as entry and exit points into and out of the state system of care for persons with a mental illness

2. Permitting DMH to purchase services from private and public providers with funds appropriated for this purpose and

requiring that the commissioner of administration promulgate rules and regulations, in consultation with the DMH director, which may include authorizing DMH to purchase technical services direct.

In the mid to late 1980s, the commissioner of administration hampered DMH efforts to develop a stable system of care for persons with a mental illness, based in large part on private community mental health centers. Throughout this period, DMH efforts to contract directly with *administrative agents*[46] without competitive bids were questioned by the state Office of Administration. This obstacle was permanently removed in 1990, when the Missouri General Assembly, working in concert with Jim Moody, the new commissioner of administration, passed legislation specifically authorizing DMH to recognize administrative agents and to contract with them directly without competitive bids.

THE BUDGET CRISIS OF 1981: SHORT- AND LONG-TERM IMPACTS

For fiscal year 1981, DMH was awarded an appropriations amount that totaled more than 10% of the state's general revenue. Halfway through that budget year, Governor Joe Teasdale was replaced by former Governor Christopher "Kit" Bond, who inherited a severe economic downturn, in great measure related to the state's prominent position in the slumping auto manufacturing industry. Shortly after taking office, Bond was forced to make massive budget cuts, with those agencies dependent on state general revenue at the greatest risk. Because these reductions could not be implemented until March, the net effect was a cut totaling one-third of the funds remaining for department operations and purchased services, spread over the last four months of the fiscal year. DMH responded by ranking client and service needs based on these four criteria [3]:

---

[46] The administrative agent approach was adapted from the concept of *exclusive contractors* proposed in NASMHPD's Partnership for Mental Health Act of 1979 and incorporated in the Mental Health Systems Act.

1. Public (including patient) protection
2. Severity of disability
3. Availability of alternate resources
4. Clinical versus ancillary services.

Highest priority was reserved for clinical services that were non-duplicative and directed toward persons who were most severely disabled, with special attention paid to situations that warranted protection of individuals or the general public. The cuts were devastating on DMH operations and contract providers. More than 1,300 department employees were laid off. To avert further lay-offs, the remaining 11,000 staff worked one day a month for no pay to the end of the fiscal year in June, a condition that affected no other state department. DMH withdrew funding for education and vocational rehabilitation programs at its state hospitals, and drastically reduced children's inpatient services. It restricted CMHC support to services for persons with acute and other serious mental illnesses, with the highest priority directed toward former mental hospital patients and persons who met the criteria for involuntary commitment. DMH's limited funding of CMHC-sponsored prevention programs was also suspended.

When fiscal year 1982 arrived on July 1, 1981, there was some financial relief. But before 12 months had elapsed, DMH officials had met with CMHC directors, advising them to gear up for more services for persons with serious and persistent mental illnesses, and less support for less seriously impaired clients. This warning proved to be painfully prophetic. For more than two decades, the state's economy would be subject to wide fluctuations. Unfortunately for DMH, its CMHC partners and the consumers they serve, in most years DMH funding as a percentage of overall state revenue would decline systematically, regardless of revenue gains or losses at the state level[47].

---

[47] For example, during the prosperous 1990s, while some agencies and practitioners serving other client groups received periodic, even annual, cost-of-living increases, such increases were routinely denied to the statewide system of CMHC administrative agents and other DMH provider groups. See also Ahr [5] Issue 1: *State funding for DMH.*

MAJOR REFORM OF COMMUNITY MENTAL HEALTH SERVICES

Statutory changes in 1980 provided DMH leadership with the opportunity to reconfigure the array and distribution of community mental health services in Missouri; the budget crisis of 1981 provided the impetus to do it soon. Beginning in spring 1981, DMH initiated four major interrelated changes in its community mental health program.

First, DMH reduced the 36 catchment areas to 26 service areas, prompting consolidation of smaller programs, especially in the central Missouri area around Jefferson City and Lake of the Ozarks, as well as in far southeast Missouri. Smaller catchment area realignments were also carried out in the metropolitan St. Louis area.

Second, DMH implemented its administrative agent initiative. Under this program, one entity within each service area was the recipient of the department's POS funding for all mental illness services provided in its designated area. Previously, DMH had entered into separate contracts with more than 50 provider agencies statewide. This new procedure reduced the number of contractors to no more than 26. State mental hospitals and the most comprehensive CMHCs were designated as DMH administrative agents in their service areas. In order for a private not-for-profit community mental health agency to be designated as an administrative agent, it was required to have a governing board comprised of local persons, to have completed a local needs assessment and plan of services for meeting identified community mental health needs, and to demonstrate a willingness to work cooperatively with other local mental health agencies to which they might be required to distribute DMH funds. In every case, local mental health agencies, including newly constituted entities in the consolidated areas, submitted applications that met these criteria, and the designations were made without challenge.

Third, DMH established a three-tier system for developing comprehensive mental health services statewide, years of rapid growth of federally funded CMHCs having resulted in service inequities across Missouri's service areas. Under the new plan, service areas were designated at one of three levels of development: core, intermediate and full service, as follows [76]:

1) Core clinics provided (or were targeted to provide):
   a) Mental health screening
   b) 24-hour-a-day emergency services (at least at the level of telephone contact)
   c) Outpatient counseling (at least at the level of two full-time counselors)
   d) Aftercare (at least at the level of a half-time physician and a budget for medication)
   e) Information and referral
   f) Case management services

2) Intermediate clinics provided (or were targeted to provide):
   a) Mental health screening
   b) 24-hour-a-day emergency services (face-to-face, when clinically indicated)
   c) Outpatient counseling
   d) Aftercare
   e) Information and referral
   f) Case management services
   g) A day program offering psychosocial rehabilitation
   h) A 24-hour-a-day residential program providing alternative living arrangements such as a group home or apartment living program

3) Full-service centers provided:
   a) Mental health screening
   b) 24-hour-a-day emergency services (face-to-face, when clinically indicated)
   c) Outpatient counseling
   d) Aftercare
   e) Information and referral
   f) Case management services
   g) A day program offering psychosocial rehabilitation
   h) A 24-hour-a-day residential program providing inpatient care in a hospital setting

A top funding priority for DMH was providing equal access to comprehensive mental health services statewide by completing the service arrays needed to designate a service area as core, intermediate or full service. Per capita funding ranges were also adopted for each of the three levels of service availability.

Finally, DMH further rationalized funding allocations by developing and implementing a methodology for standardizing the rates paid for comparable services to clinics and centers. Simply stated, for each service category, DMH ranked by price the units of services purchased from administrative agents. These unit costs were separated into four quartiles, based on price. Unit prices in the top (costliest) quartile were frozen, except through cost-of-living adjustments. Services for which the unit prices were in the lowest (least costly) quartile were carefully reviewed for quality. In every instance, the bottom price for these units was raised to the lowest rate in the second quartile, simultaneously directing these centers to upgrade the level of service they provided in this category. Thereafter, all unit costs below the cut-off point between the third and fourth quartiles (as adjusted for inflation) could be modified through a variety of means up to that cut-off point. This procedure allowed for a gradual migration of unit costs to a standard rate near the third-fourth quartiles break, which itself could be adjusted for inflation.

When Governor Bond agreed to tie POS rate increases to the rate of salary adjustments for state employees, all clinics and centers were able to realize increases similar, but not necessarily equal, to those realized by DMH operations. Ten years later, that progressive approach to funding equity would be a dim memory.

COUNTY MILL TAXES HELP SUSTAIN SOME CMHCS

In 1969, the Missouri General Assembly passed legislation that permitted residents of counties (and the freestanding City of St. Louis) to voluntarily tax themselves to develop and maintain local programs for persons with a mental illness or developmental disability. Whereas county mill taxes for developmental disabil-

184

ities services were passed in a preponderance of Missouri's counties, taxes for mental health services failed to take off. One obstacle was the requirement that all counties in a CMHC catchment area needed to authorize the tax in order for it to be levied area wide. This problem was resolved when the Missouri General Assembly passed new county mill tax legislation in 1978, permitting the passage of the tax on a county-by-county basis. Legislative sponsors and CMHC advocates pointed out the importance of county tax support to sustain CMHC operations, especially at a time when centers were reaching the limits of their federal support.

The 1978 legislation also clarified the role of DMH in the distribution of county tax funds. Specifically, the department was required to designate in its state mental health plan which entities were eligible to receive such county funds. In 1981, challenges to this requirement of the county tax statutes led Ahr to seek a formal legal opinion from Missouri Attorney General John Ashcroft. In his opinion [6], Ashcroft stated that county boards established to administer these funds shall expend them only for the following purposes of establishing or maintaining comprehensive mental health services:

(1) Providing necessary funds to establish, operate, and maintain community mental health clinics, or any comprehensive mental health services;

(2) Providing funds to supplement existing funds for the operation and maintenance of community mental health centers, mental health clinics, or any comprehensive mental health services;

(3) Purchasing any of the comprehensive mental health services from community mental health centers, mental health clinics, and other public facilities or not-for-profit corporations which are designated by the department. (Emphasis supplied in the opinion.)

This opinion highlighted that the legislature had assigned to DMH the duty to designate recipients of the county funds, in order to promote coordination and minimize duplication of services. Based on this understanding of the law, DMH officials, including Dr. Robert Jones, director of DMH's Division of Comprehensive Psychiatric Services [75], set out to designate DMH's administrative agents as the eligible recipients of county mill tax funds.

GREAT RIVERS MENTAL HEALTH SERVICES

By 1983, one major part of the state's mental health landscape remained relatively untouched by these improvements: St. Louis County. With a population nearing one million, Missouri's most populous county was still being served by an outreach clinic from St. Louis State Hospital. The ready supply of mental health agencies and practitioners provided DMH with the opportunity to install a radically new service delivery system. According to DMH officials, there were 300 mental health providers in St. Louis County, and it did not make sense to them to create the 301st. The serious limitation on available funds[48] also precluded the establishment of a conventional community mental health center. The resolution was a new form of community mental health agency modeled on the highly successful St. Louis Regional Center for the Developmentally Disabled, another DMH operation. This new entity was named Great Rivers Mental Health Services.

Under the leadership of Bonnie DiFranco[49], a longtime DMH employee, Great Rivers negotiated contracts with community mental health agencies and private practitioners to provide services for the agency's clients. Great Rivers was responsible for all aspects of the clients' case management: initial screening and intake, treatment planning, follow-up care (including changes in clients' care plans as warranted). Developed in an era when the term *managed care* had not yet been coined, Great Rivers pioneered managing the care of clients for whom it provided few

---

[48] St. Louis County was receiving only 40% of the statewide per-capita average.

[49] For more information on the "Great Rivers model," see the *Missouri First-Person Interviews* with Bonnie DiFranco [pp. 199-207] and Diane McFarland [pp. 209-215].

direct services. The success of this model can be measured by its direct replication in St. Louis City, and indirectly in North Kansas City, where it served as a prototype for that revitalized CMHC operation. Changes in reimbursement patterns changed the mix of purchased to provided services, and Great Rivers was transferred to BJC HealthCare in St. Louis along with St. Louis Mental Health Center and DMH's outpatient program in Park Hills[50], Missouri.

THE ROLE OF ATYPICALS

With the advent of psychotropic medications, persons with a mental illness formerly destined to a lifetime course of treatment in a mental hospital were able to be discharged from hospitals, and in some cases not be hospitalized at all. But the first generation of antipsychotic medications had unpleasant side effects, like dry mouth, stiffness and trembling, and patients often stopped using them. In 1989, Clozaril (Clozapine) entered the market, and was soon hailed as a major breakthrough in the treatment of schizophrenia. Other atypicals[51] followed: Risperdal (Risperidone) in 1994, and Zyprexa (Olanzapine) in 1996. Seroquel (Quetiapine), Geodon (Ziprasidone) and Abilify (Ariprazole) are recent entries.

According to *New York Times* reporter Erica Goode [42].

> The drugs appeared so successful that doctors began prescribing them for other things, not only for other psychotic illnesses, like manic depression, but also for Alzheimer's, personality disorders and non-psychotic depression ... More than 15 million prescriptions were written last year for the two leading drugs alone, Zyprexa and Risperdal, industry figures show.

---

[50] BJC BH serves Iron, St. Francois and Washington counties in southeast Missouri.

[51] According to Goode [42]:
European researchers who had stumbled upon the drug years before described it as "atypical" because even at very high doses, it did not produce the stiffness, trembling and other Parkinson's-like symptoms commonly seen in patients taking older antipsychotics like Haldol.

Goode reported on her interview with Dr. Joseph Parks, DMH medical director and president of NASMHPD's medical directors' council. Speaking about three atypical antipsychotics, Zyprexa, Risperdal and Seroquel, he said, "They are good medications and they seriously help a lot of people. I would not want to give up any of them." Consumers and their families agree wholeheartedly with Parks.

SHIFT TO MEDICAID

In the 1980s and early 1990s[52], DMH began to look toward Medicaid as a revenue source to adjust for declining state tax dollars. In order to position itself for this funding stream, DMH created the CPR program. Designed to assist persons with a serious and persistent mental illness to remain in the community for much longer periods of time without being hospitalized, a CPR was required to offer the following services directly or through affiliation:

1. Intake and annual evaluations
2. Crisis intervention and resolution
3. Medication services
4. Consultation services
5. Medication administration
6. Community support
7. Psychosocial rehabilitation.

CMHCs that offered all of those components were certified to be CPR providers and were able to bill Medicaid for these services. For many centers, however, this strategy placed them more firmly on a path away from serving a broad array of community members with DMH funds and closer to primarily, almost exclusively, serving Medicaid eligible persons with serious and persistent mental illnesses.

---

[52] For additional information about DMH during the period from 1986 to 2003, see the *Missouri First-Person Interviews* with Diane McFarland (pp. 209-215) and Dorn Schuffman (pp. 223-230).

Services for children and youth, less well-developed and distributed than adult services, followed a more direct route to Medicaid initiatives targeted for those with a serious emotional disturbance. Early experiences with a "prescription team" composed of representatives of state child-serving agencies set the stage for the introduction of Missouri's 503 demonstration program. This program was designed to enable children with a severe emotional disturbance to attain the following four primary goals:

1. Remain with their families, if they can remain safely and it is in the child's best interest.
2. Receive any indicated out-of-home treatment for as brief a time as possible, in the least restrictive setting consistent with effective services, and in as close proximity as possible to the child's usual residence.
3. Attend and make academic progress in school.
4. Behave in a lawful manner, not commit crimes, and not be incarcerated.

The 503 demonstration documented [8] the effectiveness of a targeted case management approach on reducing costly institutional and other out-of-home placements for children and youth. This experience served as the basis of a statewide expansion of targeted case management paid for by Medicaid. A collateral development was the establishment of Families First teams around the state for children and youth with serious emotional disturbances. These programs were made a part of the regular offerings of DMH's administrative agents statewide [90].

THE PRIVATIZATION OF STATE-OPERATED CMHCS

The process by which DMH divested itself of its own CMHC operations took place in two, somewhat unrelated, steps. In the first step, outpatient and other ambulatory care programs at state institutions were separated into new state-run agencies. In St. Louis, the DMH-operated ambulatory programs at St. Louis State Hospital and Malcolm Bliss were spun out into the St. Louis

Mental Health Center, a replica of Great Rivers. The ambulatory programs of Western Missouri and Mid-MO were transferred to Central Kansas City (CKC) and Heart of Missouri mental health centers, respectively. Outpatient services at the remaining state hospitals were de-coupled, in some cases to existing CMHCs. The primary rationale for establishing new state CMHCs was to better standardize ambulatory care operations across the state, making available in each service area community mental health programs of comparable mission. Privatization was built on this base.

In the beginning, privatization was proposed as a pilot project involving Great Rivers and St. Louis Mental Health Center. Set in the context of a re-inventing government initiative, one of its objectives was to make all of the state CMHC operations private. However, dramatic changes in payment mechanisms for mental health services[53] brought about by the move to managed care arrangements and increased reliance on Medicaid, accelerated and enlarged the privatization process.

These changes worked against state CMHCs, and in some ways in favor of private CMHCs. For example, private centers were more flexible in their program offerings, staffing options and contracting opportunities. Revenue generated by private centers was returned to these service providers for program improvements and expansion; revenue earned by DMH was returned to the state's general fund for possible, but not guaranteed, reinvestment in DMH operations.

From the perspective of DMH, the best interests of the state and its clients would be served by finding private sector partners who could take optimum advantage of the funding strategies available for mental health care. Concern about the futures of state employees demanded a request-for-proposal process that assured them job security for at least one year. These and other require-ments helped set the stage for the state centers to be privatized into large hospital systems: CKC to Truman Medical Center; Heart of

---

[53] Especially MC+, the state's managed care strategy for providing services to Medicaid eligible children.

Missouri to the University of Missouri Health Care; and Great Rivers, St. Louis Mental Health and Park Hills (previously spun off from the state hospital in Farmington) to BJC HealthCare.

University Behavioral Health Services

The wisdom of this approach became readily apparent. State-operated adult outpatient services were privatized in the area once tended by Mid-MO on June 1, 1997, and incorporated into University of Missouri Health Care where it now functions under the name University Behavioral Health Services (UBH). The children's outpatient programs were transferred to UBH on February 1, 2003.

Through leveraging and a more efficient business approach, UBH has tripled the level of service provided under DMH management (Mid-MO and later Heart of Missouri mental health centers) with special emphasis on the development of services for children and clients with co-occurring disorders. Technology has allowed more efficient and timely delivery of psychiatric services through the development of a telehealth network which connects the eleven UBH clinics. These enhancements have been achieved with essentially the same level of funding as was available prior to privatization. According to UBH Director Dr. Bruce Horwitz [53]:

> I think DMH could see that the CMHC model would give them more bang for their buck and, in our case, it succeeded. The key here was going from fixed funding to a fee-for-service contract which necessitated increased productivity and efficiency to achieve a positive margin (something the other CMHCs had been doing all along). The ability to leverage funds and retain revenue helped support expansion of services. There is nothing like fee-for-service to motivate providers!

Truman Medical Center Behavioral Health

Privatization has also proven to be a boon to the sponsor organizations and the community at large. In Kansas City, CKC brought a unique product line to Truman Medical Center. Truman top management recognized that behavioral health was not an area where their health system had internal expertise and they structured this addition in a way that embraced the skills and talents of the CKC leadership team. According to COO Marsha Morgan [80]:

> I was immediately made a member of the TMC executive team, and our operations remained separate from the hospitals' departments. I believe that this decision was a key factor to the success and ease with which we privatized. We came to the table as equals; we were not buried in a hospital department. Our billings were able to be processed, and general accounting occurred outside of the huge and different hospital structure.

Two years after privatization, Network Rehabilitation Services for People with Serious Mental Illnesses merged with Truman Behavioral Health. This organization brought complementary services to the Truman array, which now offers vocational/employment services, a clubhouse psychosocial rehabilitation program, consumer-run social programs (evening and weekend services, a drop-in center at the homeless building and an art program) and homeless outreach services, in addition to the core CMHC services.

BJC Behavioral Health Community Services

Not all consolidations were completed as easily as the one implemented by CKC and Truman Medical Center. According to Diane McFarland[54], across the state in St. Louis and Park Hills it took a

---

[54] Ms. McFarland is director of the Division of Comprehensive Psychiatric Services. In her *Missouri First-Person Interview* [pp. 209-215], she recounts the early history of Great Rivers Mental Health Services and the St. Louis Mental Health Center.

while for BJC and the former Great Rivers Mental Health Services, St. Louis Mental Health Center and Park Hills CMHC to find the right niche. Mark Stansberry [97], executive director of BJC BH, tells how things have worked out:

> The leadership of BJC HealthCare is firmly committed to the services provided by the community mental health center. Following its placement in a separate corporation within the BJC HealthCare structure, BJC BH enjoys a certain amount of autonomy in its service delivery system and is viewed as a key component in BJC HealthCare's community outreach objectives. BJC BH also benefits from this arrangement by being able to draw upon the infrastructure capabilities of the parent organization.

EMERGING REGIONALIZATION

Since 1997, changes in the level and sources of funds for CMHC operations have promoted regionalization of services, within the context of a center's responsibility for a defined service area, in three primary arenas. The first was the voluntary mergers of smaller centers into the Pathways Behavioral Health Care partnership.

The second was the creation of the crisis access system. Recognizing the need for higher quality responses to consumer emergencies, DMH launched a new 24-hour crisis response system known as Access Crisis Intervention (ACI). The goals of ACI are:

1. To provide immediate response, intervention and referral for persons experiencing mental health crisis on a 24-hour, 7-day-a-week basis whether in a rural, urban or metropolitan area.
2. To respond to crisis by providing community-based intervention in the least restrictive environment, e.g., home, school.
3. To avert the need for hospitalization to the greatest extent possible.
4. To stabilize persons in crisis and refer them to appropriate services to regain an optimal level of functioning.

5. To mobilize and link individuals with services, resources and supports needed for ongoing care following a crisis, including natural support networks.

These goals are achieved through a sophisticated program of telephone triage and intervention, backed up by face-to-face crisis stabilization from mobile teams throughout the state. Immediate respite and inpatient services are available, if deemed necessary, and next-day appointments for less acute situations allow consumers to receive mental health services in a timely manner. Funding constraints precluded each CMHC from developing independent crisis systems that met DMH's new, higher standards. As a result, CMHCs pooled their resources to implement the new service.

Third, these early experiences with joint ventures helped pave the way for other cooperative projects, especially activities designed to deal with state-sponsored and other managed care initiatives. In the greater Kansas City area, CMHCs and other mental health organizations[55] jointly created CommCare to deal with crisis access and managed care requirements. Similarly, the CMHCs in the greater St. Louis area[56] created BHR to deal with crisis access. Both of these enterprises have branched out into other mental health related product lines.

SYSTEM REDESIGN

Each of these changes to the community-based services system in Missouri was a logical adjustment of a maturing administrative agent system to circumstances not foreseen when it was first installed in the early 1980s. At the end of the 1990s, however, another proposed initiative took direct aim at the state's system of community-based mental health care and threatened its viability.

---

[55] CommCare is a joint venture of the six Kansas City CMHCs, Pathways Community Behavioral Healthcare, North Central Missouri Mental Health Center, Family Guidance Center and Kansas City Community Center.

[56] They are: Crider Center, COMTREA, Hopewell Center and BJC BH.

Beginning in 1996, DMH leadership systematically pursued a program of public discussion and policymaking referred to as *system redesign* [77]. Intended to develop the department's preferred approach for the financing, management and evaluation of services for some Missourians who required publicly funded psychiatric and substance abuse treatment and supports, the system redesign effort followed prior unsuccessful efforts to introduce for-profit managed care practices in its operations. Facilitated by out-of-state consultants, the direction of the system redesign effort was met with caution by mental health advocacy and provider organizations. By July 1998, representatives of these organizations[57] and other mental health professionals and private citizens presented a joint statement to the DMH System Redesign Steering Committee. Over the next 14 months, the Federation of Missouri Advocates for Mental Health and Substance Abuse Services (Federation) would prepare and present three more critiques of DMH's unfolding system redesign proposals, culminating in the publication of *Reasonable Expectations for the Design and Operation of a System of Publicly Funded Psychiatric and Substance Abuse Treatment Services and Supports* [31].

The Federation's opposition to the major tenets of DMH's position was based on two primary factors:

1. Since the early 1980s, DMH and its administrative agent partners had been implementing a system of care that was based on principles of eligibility, access, utilization and cost that would later be referred to as *managed care.*
2. For-profit managed care approaches in other states had failed when they were applied to public sector settings, and under then current funding arrangements, these approaches could

---

[57] Initial signatories to this series of documents included representatives of the Missouri Mental Health Consumer Network, Missouri Statewide Parent Advisory Network, Mental Health Association of Greater St. Louis, Depressive and Manic Depressive Association and NAMI of St. Louis. By September 1999, when public comments on the last of its system redesign formal proposals were due at the DMH, the list of signatories had grown to include more than a dozen organizations, and the combined group named itself the Federation of Missouri Advocates for Mental Health and Substance Abuse Services.

only succeed in Missouri by severely limiting access to publicly funded mental health care[58].

Service and financing improvements installed by DMH in the early 1980s set in place a managed care approach that predates contemporary managed care applications, and was embraced by CMHCs. In the DMH methodology, the best-qualified provider of services in each geographic (service) area was selected to provide a predetermined array of services to a specific population group, based on geography. Funding allocations for these service providers, known as administrative agents, were arrived at by two means.

First, DMH set overall allocations based on the level of service provided (core, intermediate or full service). Second, reimbursement levels were set based on a plan of service (i.e., number of units to be offered) tied to negotiated rates for each service component. Historic differences in rates were gradually collapsed by holding the top rates relatively constant, while allowing low- and mid-level rates to migrate to a common flat-rate level over time. Cost and quality controls were maintained by DMH. Local variations in service requirements were promoted to DMH by citizen boards of directors, while regional coordination was achieved through the active participation of regional citizen advisory councils. Over time, the state's system of mental health care would stabilize to at least the level of intermediate clinics. In an environment of funding stability, administrative agents were better able to leverage state funds for additional services not paid for by DMH. By the start of the 1990s, this approach had been altered by other contractual and funding mechanisms, but remained the basis for future DMH-CMHC partnerships.

---

[58] It is important to note that CMHCs in Missouri have routinely implemented managed care principles. The Federation's concern was with the strategies employed by for-profit managed care companies to assure a profit for shareholders. Pamela Hyde, DMH's primary system redesign consultant, has pointed out [57] that: "While cost containment is the aim of health care reform (of which managed care is a part), profit is the driving force behind the interest of private companies in becoming players in the heretofore largely public sector of behavioral health care."

By the late 1990s, there were several highly publicized failures [16, 52, 69, 91, 96, 100] and critiques [73, 74] of for-profit managed care approaches in the public sector. These failures and the related history of uncompensated care being provided to publicly supported clients by community-based mental health agencies in many states demonstrated the invalidity of the basic economic assumptions on which these risk-based or capitated payment systems were built. Simply stated, the risk hypothesis in health care financing presumes that, if the party that assumes risk prevents illness to the greatest extent possible and provides just the right treatments to just the right (i.e., eligible) persons in just the right dosage to achieve the minimally acceptable outcomes, there should be enough money left in the contract with the funding organization to provide for a profit. If there is no possibility of profit (i.e., if the base level of funding is inadequate), then the risk-assuming party is predestined to fail. The groups who would be at the greatest risk if private (i.e., for-profit) organizations fail are the children and youth with a serious emotional disturbance or substance abuse problem and adults with a serious and persistent mental illness or substance abuse problem – the very consumers DMH has been funded to serve [55].

For at least the past 35 years in Missouri, costs for treating consumers of DMH-funded services have been only partially borne by DMH. Additional costs have been borne by local not-for-profit agencies through cost shifting from private sector clients, local taxes, fund raising and doing without. Consumers have also had to do without. While reliable data on un-served needs is difficult to obtain, publicly funded mental health agencies throughout Missouri have long maintained waiting lists for their consumers and have been required to provide partial or substitute services (e.g., group for individual therapies) because of a lack of the resources needed to provide the most cost beneficial services. Other consumers have simply not received services because they have not been available to them.

Because of the chronic under-financing of DMH-funded services, even for a more limited range of DMH target populations, DMH would have been unable to institute a fully capitated financing mechanism for its consumers until there was adequate funding (state or federal) to pay for it. The Federation argued correctly that until DMH was able to secure adequate funding to meet the minimal requirements of the risk hypothesis, it should be precluded from implementing a fully capitated financing approach for its consumers. Rather, DMH should work to establish enhanced public-private partnerships with its certified providers of mental health services. Within months, the *Show Me System Redesign* initiative set below the horizon.

By 2001, twenty years after the inauguration of the administrative agent approach, this community-based system of care had been tested once again, and once again prevailed[59]. Spawned in the spirit of the national Mental Health Systems Act of 1980 and designed in the state Omnibus Mental Health Act of the same year, it was installed during the state's financial crisis of 1981. Reinforced by a critical statutory change in 1990, this approach was expanded to include newly formed state outpatient centers that were privatized in 1997. With the assistance of other not-for-profit organizations and advocates for persons with an emotional disturbance or mental illness, the integrity of the CMHC provider system as an agent of DMH was forcefully defended in 1999. Budget reductions in the late 1990s and early 2000s have further narrowed the gap between CMHCs and state operations, as has DMH Director Dorn Schuffman, a veteran of more than two-dozen years of working collaboratively with Missouri's CMHCs.

---

[59] The status of administrative agents was addressed again in August 2003. In an audit of DMH's Division of Comprehensive Psychiatric Services [79] Missouri Auditor Claire McCaskill, stated:

> The division's contractors offer a continuum of therapeutic and treatment services for state residents diagnosed with mental illness. Allowed by statute, these service providers are considered the gatekeepers of Missouri's mental health delivery system.

MISSOURI FIRST-PERSON INTERVIEW WITH:

BONNIE DIFRANCO

Bonnie DiFranco MSW, LCSW, from St. Louis, Missouri, worked for the Department of Mental Health from 1973 to 2000. She has had extensive experience with adult and child mental health programs. Ms. DiFranco worked for ten years in community services and inpatient children's services as a social worker and a unit manager. In 1983, she became the director of Great Rivers Mental Health Services, a state-run community mental health program in St. Louis County, Missouri, where she remained until 1996. Ms. DiFranco completed her career with the department as the acting CEO of Metropolitan St. Louis Psychiatric Center, an acute care hospital. Currently, Ms. DiFranco is engaged in private consulting.

I started my career in 1973, right out of graduate social work school at what was then Malcolm Bliss Mental Health Center. In 1974, I was working as a social worker in the traveling clinic at St. Charles where there was a rather extensive program for children and adults. For the adult services, they had at least two full-time psychiatrists, two social workers, and psychology interns who would come out and work with some of the therapy clients. They also had support staff. In the children's program, which was only one day a week, we had two psychiatrists and two social workers. It was almost a full-time outreach clinic. Malcolm Bliss made quite a commitment to this program.

I worked with the traveling clinic until I went to what was then the Youth Center, the new children's hospital. I was a unit manager with the Youth Center and then went to St. Louis State Hospital to be the unit manager of outpatient services. That is when I got involved with all of the traveling clinics. At the time, both Malcolm Bliss and St. Louis State Hospital had catchment areas for traveling clinics. State Hospital tended to go south and went to Washington, Missouri, which was a true traveling clinic except for a full-time clerical. They had services maybe two days a week. There was a program in Hillsboro, which was in the Jefferson County health department, and that program ran several days a week. There was an outreach clinic in Kinlock, which actually had six or seven staff who were housed full time, and a psychiatrist would travel back and forth to that program. There was the full-time St. Louis County program which was five days a week with a staff of close to thirty individuals. Bliss had a one-day-a-week program in Troy and Warrenton.

The communities were very protective of these programs. We regularly attended community meetings; we were very involved in the community council and would attend the community council meetings in St. Charles. We were quite involved with the social service agencies. It was a viable entity and it really didn't feel like we were intruders in any way, shape or form. The programs got a number of referrals; we probably had more referrals than we could ever handle. St. Louis County, Hillsboro, St. Charles, were really viable entities where the community was quite involved.

The state of Missouri had the interest to create community programs and to give the services to the community rather than the community actually begging for these programs. COMTREA was a contracted substance abuse program in Jefferson County and had been in business for quite some time. Steve Huss was the CEO at that time. They had a very active board, and we negotiated with that board, moving the services and actual dollars to those programs from the budgets of the two state facilities.

It was not difficult to find people to work in those clinics. First of all, they were well organized; people came for their appointments. You did not have quite the various crisis problems you had walking into the Malcolm Bliss outpatient program or the St. Louis State Hospital outpatient program. Things worked primarily like a therapy clinic. The parents and families were highly motivated to come for treatment; there was a lot of work with the schools. That was probably the thing that I loved the most; we would actually sit in classrooms with the teachers and observe the children and help the teacher as to how to deal with some of the behavioral issues.

For a while, in St. Charles, we actually had a special education specialist, Charlene Schultz, who came out one day a week and spent time working in the schools with the teachers. It was a very dynamic place and we had a lot of bright interns and it was a place people wanted to go.

What was really exciting about the traveling clinics was the development of the psychiatric component for both adults and children in Jefferson County and the actual development of the board and the leadership of the St. Charles community to pull a very viable board together. Malcolm Bliss's superintendent, Dr. Kathleen Smith, and I would go to St. Charles and meet with the interested citizens. That was a pretty exciting venture for that community to have that kind of commitment, and obviously Jane Crider was a key in that.

The biggest issue in Jefferson County was that all the staff members had been trained in substance abuse services. They had a tremendous history and commitment to that service, so to turn around a group of people to want to provide the psychiatric services was a challenge. I think that Steve Huss provided a tremendous amount of leadership in making this work. It was in their site in Hillsboro, and his main site was in Festus. He needed to communicate to make sure there were enough services throughout the county for everybody. He was really very good in making this happen. It took some time to change the focus.

At the time probably the biggest discrepancy in terms of fairness and equity in the state was in St. Louis County which had about 25% of the population at that time but did not have its own mental health center. It was an extension of St. Louis State Hospital. Many of the areas had taken advantage of the community mental health center movement, but St. Louis County never did. The county had made a commitment to an outpatient children's program, but that was pretty much it.

Paul Ahr was DMH director and he made a very strong commitment to develop a program in St. Louis County. DMH worked with area legislators. There was tremendous interest in what was to become Great Rivers Mental Health Services. There was a very targeted campaign to really help people understand why this needed to be done. There were some key legislative leaders like Representatives Sue Shear and Laurie Donovan who were also very important in its development.

Dr. Ahr established a very different model than what was going on in Missouri at that time. Given the way St. Louis County was situated, with a huge population of about a million people and about 505 square miles, it would have been very costly to put money in bricks and mortar and establish a number of sites in St. Louis County. He presented a concept of a case management broker model where there would be a central site and case managers to oversee the consumers; but all of the services would be contracted out to local private psychiatrists, psychologists and any other service entities that were needed by the agency. The beauty of it was that individuals who were coming for state services could actually go to private offices in their home territory. The agency could contract with all kinds of specialists, giving us a tremendous opportunity to get a variety of contractors across the county.

It was an extremely hard sell to get started. First of all, there was limited funding and everybody was pressuring to have services. There was a limit to the number of dollars and so I had to start in one area first. We needed to implement the model so we could sell it to other providers. I actually had to make cold calls. I went from one hospital to another and literally knocked on doors and went in and charmed the receptionist to either let me talk to the doctors at that time or to get an appointment. When I tried to talk to people, they kept saying that they were not going to deal with the state; they were thinking of Medicaid. It was important to show them the actual contract and show them the system. I would also send them information – send them some samples of what we would be doing so that they would have time to read it.

The Eastern Missouri Psychiatric Association let me send information to its members. The psychiatrists were the toughest to get. Psychologists and social workers always wanted other business, but the psychiatrists were the hardest sell. Eventually we started getting psychiatrists. They would refer us to other psychiatrists and then it came to the point where psychiatrists would be calling, asking to be providers. In this model we had varying rates based upon a provider's specialty or expertise. We could negotiate different rates with providers, which was really excellent because there were some psychiatrists who were tremendously valuable to the program. There were two other important issues with contracting services. One was that you could buy varying pieces of a clinician's time. Second, the psychiatrists had to provide the after hours on call as part of their responsibilities to their consumers just like their private practice. Consumers were given the number of their private psychiatrists where they could call them after hours. Providers would invoice us and then it would be checked by the case manager to make sure that the information was accurate. As far as compliance, we would crosscheck with consumers to make sure they were seen; we would do a random sample of consumers to make sure they saw the psychiatrist on that date. We only paid for services provided, not for no-shows.

The original staff came from the outpatient clinics, which did not work out too well. They were primarily people who were therapists, who might just do individual therapy or groups. As staff left and as we were able to get more money, we started hiring master's-level case managers who really wanted to do case management.

Initially, there were not children's services at Great Rivers because of the financial issues of the agency. Linda Roebuck decided to place the St. Louis County 503 program at Great Rivers, and that is when the kick-off of children's services started. The 503 program was a wraparound program; it was a partnership arrangement. The program was based on the concept of all of the children's agencies coming together at the table and working with the high-end high-risk children to try to reduce the duplication of services. The concept was that every children's agency, education, social services, juvenile court, etc., would put in money at the table and would together use this money to provide services for the children. Basically, it was the leaders of these programs who would get together each month, and they would actually staff children and decide which children would go into the 503 program.

We were able to do targeted case management in a way that would make people proud. Each targeted case manager only had ten children and families. The beauty of the model of 503 was actually giving the parents the right to make the decision from an array of services of what they thought their child needed. I think that it was more than the agencies coming together; it was those initial targeted case managers who philosophically understood so well how to work with those families and to give those parents the power to really dictate how services went and really worked.

At that time, everything was operating on the broker model. There were not any other services provided other than the targeted case management. The broker model continued to thrive until the Medicaid rehabilitation option and children's program; that is what eventually changed the agency from a total broker model to having to provide some services directly. When we ran the numbers, we could not afford to offer the Medicaid services, especially the children's Medicaid program, at the reimbursement rate, unless we provided services directly. We provided the community support services directly in concert with the case management services. But as far as some of the other psychiatric service choices, we just could not afford to purchase all of them. Reimbursement rates, the time factor, the cost of the brokering, the cost of the communication required, and all of the signatures, etc., that were required, were all factors. We just could not do it, so we brought in psychiatrists who would primarily do a Medicaid program for children's services and some adult services.

It was a hard shift for me; it was a tremendously hard shift for me because I was running two models. It was much more difficult to control whom came through the door in terms of expertise available. You could no longer offer people the expertise that we were able to offer before. A number of the psychiatrists did not want to deal with some of the issues of the Medicaid program and all of the paperwork, etc., involved in it. In the adult program we were using primarily private psychiatrists; in the children's program we had to go totally to a staff model. That was the one that was financially unfeasible otherwise.

When I left in 1996, two-thirds of the Great Rivers operations were still utilizing a broker model. The broker model still exists with the new entity, which was privatized in 1997; they have a large number of contractors and they have someone who is specifically in charge of contract services and negotiating and developing contracts.

John Twiehaus believed that hospitals should be in the business of running hospitals and that outpatient programs were stepchildren of hospitals and never would grow and never would have strength unless they were pulled out and either given to a community mental health center or developed. So he decided to create in the City of St. Louis a replica of Great Rivers because he really believed that this was a very successful model. I was pulled from Great Rivers for a year and went to the city. I worked for one year in closing both outpatient programs, looking for an operation, a building, looking at what staff were needed. Diane McFarland was the first director of St. Louis Mental Health Center.

RESPONSIBILITY FOR A SPECIFIED POPULATION: Great Rivers was responsible for the residents of St. Louis County and the individuals, a child or adult, coming out of the hospitals that resided in St. Louis County. For those who were hospitalized we provided the aftercare.

PREVENTION AND EARLY INTERVENTION: We were never able to do what would be technically called prevention. However, for the children's program we would target children and provide services to children who were in families where the parents had schizophrenia. We tried to work to give them as many services as possible and offer the parents respite and those types of things.

TREATING PEOPLE IN THEIR HOME COMMUNITIES: We tried to prevent further hospitalization by working really strongly through case management. We tried to look at what caused the hospitalization and what we could do to prevent that from occurring in the future.

CONTINUUM OF CARE: We had a very large continuum of care and the finest medications. We were always in trouble for having such a big pharmacy budget because we felt we needed to have on our formulary the best medicine that was available. There was a full continuum of care. At the start, the DMH director created a computerized assessment system and every individual that walked through the doors of Great Rivers went to the computer and was assisted in completing a series of questions which resulted in us getting a baseline of what some of the key problems were. We addressed not only their illness and alcohol or substance abuse, but also loneliness and isolation. We would develop a global assessment functioning (GAF) score and from there we would track that GAF score. We had a wellness level towards the end. The last three or four years we had about 70-80 people on a wellness level who had actually sustained a consistent GAF score for at least one year. There was also a symptom checklist that clients completed.

MULTIDISCIPLINARY TEAMS: I never had paraprofessional staff that I worked with. It was kind of prior to some of the things with peer support, peer specialist. We did not have paraprofessionals other than the respite workers.

LINKAGES WITH OTHER ORGANIZATIONS: In the children's program, we were heavily linked programmatically to a number of the children's agencies. Part of the model of community is to work very closely not only with families but also with some of the community agencies that people need as support in their lives – everything from nurses coming into their homes to social services, etc.

FISCAL AND PROGRAMMATIC ACCOUNTABILITY: We were a state of Missouri program so we were fiscally responsible to the legislature as well as to DMH and to our own utilization management model philosophy. We wanted to use our dollars to stretch and to provide services that were most needed.

CITIZEN PARTICIPATION: We had advisory boards. I can only speak to the advisory board at Great Rivers and I don't know that I could have survived without the advisory board. The board was made up of persons who were highly respected in the community. For example, we had as board members Dr. Ray Knowles, a prominent physician in St. Louis; Nick Franchot and Jerry Zafft who had been members of the Missouri Mental Health Commission; and Dr. Ahr, the former director of DMH who established Great Rivers. It was all the things a community board needed to be in terms of protecting the agency, making sure its reputation was a good one and making sure the right decisions were made. It was a very, very committed board.

Diane McFarland currently serves as director of the Division of Comprehensive Services for the Missouri Department of Mental Health. She received her master's degree in social work from Washington University in St. Louis. Her career in community mental health started in 1983 when she became one of the original case managers at Great Rivers Mental Health Services, helping to establish the broker model of service. Ms. McFarland later served as quality assurance specialist and then became the executive director of the newly developed St. Louis Mental Health Center in 1989. Her latest former position was as executive director of BJC Behavioral Health, which comprised the merged operations of Great Rivers, St. Louis MHC and Park Hills Mental Health Services, which were privatized under BJC HealthCare in 1997. She lives in St. Louis with her husband, John, and her three sons, Ryan, Cory and Trevor.

I got started in 1980 at Malcolm Bliss Mental Health Center as a social worker in the outpatient clinic. I got laid off within about six months, went back to school and got my master's degree and started up again at Great Rivers as one of the original case managers. I started up the transition from doing direct services to contracted services. We were still developing the providers, so as we developed them, we transitioned the clients to the providers and started up the authorization process and the monitoring process. The job of getting the providers was Bonnie DiFranco's. We started with a few psychosocial providers; psychiatrists started building and we got a lot of psychotherapy providers: psychologists and social workers. We controlled the assessment and treatment planning process. Bonnie established systems for regular provider reporting. I was acting director of Great Rivers while Bonnie set up St. Louis Mental Health Center in 1989. That entailed finding a building and finding providers. When she came back to Great Rivers, I went over to St. Louis Mental Health Center. It is exactly the same model as that at Great Rivers.

Privatization and splitting the outpatient services at state facilities from their inpatient programs were two separate steps. They were two very distinct processes. First, they separated the community-based services from the inpatient services in the state facilities. Privatization occurred in 1997. The original plan was just to do a pilot with Great Rivers and St. Louis Mental Health Center and spin them off into a single not-for-profit, but then they went statewide and all the state community mental health agencies were included and it went to a request for proposal process, not just a spin-off. When it was a pilot project, it was part of DMH's re-inventing government activities. It was intended to get a more uniform system for the community services – not to have seven state centers and the rest not-for-profit. The administrative agent system was strong, and this was a way to strengthen that and get the state out of direct service. My personal opinion is that John Twiehaus built on the administrative agent system very well.

What was going to be the pilot was designed to see what happens when state programs are privatized, especially the broker model, since Great Rivers and St. Louis Mental Health Center were on the broker model. Managed care coming into play with MC+ was what really drove the decision to go statewide and get all the outpatient services so that they could contract and compete, not knowing where MC+ and managed care were going to go in the future. A big part of it was that if the state provided a reimbursable service, the revenue went into the general fund, whereas if a private provider did it, the money went directly back into building the provider's program. I also think that at that time, the state was not ready to go into managed care contracting with state facilities. I see the spinning off of the outpatient units and privatization as a natural evolution of what we had before.

There were two bidders on Great Rivers and St. Louis Mental Health Center. The financial and reserve requirements severely limited who could bid on the RFPs. It was going to have to be a fairly financially stable and large organization to make this work.

Five state outpatient operations were bid out. CKC went to Truman Medical Center; Heart of Missouri went to the University of Missouri Health Care; Great Rivers, St. Louis Mental Health and Park Hills went to BJC.

From a service perspective, the opportunities after privatization are greater. In looking back, the infrastructure transition posed some challenges. We basically unplugged from the state and we plugged into a very large entity with a very different infrastructure. Information systems and the operations placement in governance and structure are the two areas that took a great deal of time to work out. With Truman Medical Center, Central Kansas City got organizationally structured very well. In the case of Great Rivers/ St. Louis Mental Health/Park Hills, it took a couple of legal changes in operations and organizational structure to get to that. I think that it was because of size and the fact that the system was going through other operations changes and a lot of growth at the time.

On leaving BJC, I felt the service model was successfully integrated and became much stronger after privatization. Some of the consolidation, although it took a very long time, strongly supported it. We had some extremely dedicated staff from the three centers. They came together in some very new roles, stuck with it and brought the three centers into a cohesive whole. Terri Gilbert, Karen Miller, Jamie Zacharias, Emily Riley and Jackie Gilliland, to name a few, are some of the most mission-driven people I know and that's what made it work. I was glad I had supportive management at BJC. From the point of view of a health system, there's not a lot of logic to operating a broker model mental health system, especially across other health systems. Also, as an administrative agent for the state, it's a non-competitive model set within a competitive environment. We were initially under Betty Leventhal, the patient care services director at Barnes-Jewish Hospital. That was just an interim structure, but she was phenomenal. She brought it all in and helped get us set up and settled in a very new environment. She was such an advocate for clients, which suited us well. She worked very hard and continued to advocate for us when we spun off into a separate legal structure under the managed care arm of the system. Peter Ambrose was in charge and provided a lot of support then. When that division was phased out, we made another change and went under Joan Magruder, who was part of the BJC senior executive team. She was determined to help us make that final transition successful and was the key to us finally getting fully plugged into the system the way we should be. I'd say another real champion at the system level, throughout all the changes, was Ed Stiften, the chief financial officer who said, "How does this fit; what does this really do?" and risked spinning us off into a separate 501(c)(3) under BJC HealthCare. His support and mentoring went beyond mere financials.

Comprehensive psychiatric rehabilitation came into play as a Medicaid program at the time that St. Louis Mental Health Center came into existence. The MC+ system for kids and some adults was set up and run by an entirely different system. It was a risk to CMHCs that did not operate as direct service providers, which flew in the face of the Great Rivers and SLMHC design. You either had to be a direct service provider or you had to partner with one and see if you could bid to become the managed care organization.

The 24-hour crisis access system was another major milestone. Everybody was given some flexibility of how to set up their 24-hour access system. That was coming on at the same time as managed care, and some people tried to organize together such as CommCare and BHR and become a managed care company and a 24-hour crisis access service. BHR chose not to pursue the managed care option. However, it did offer 24-hour access to the managed care organizations under contract. BHR actually went live the day MC+ started on the sixth floor of our downtown office. We set up some desks and hooked up phones, and clinical staff from all five centers rotated through to man the calls. I'll never forget some of the staff who traveled miles at night only to arrive for their "extra duty" and literally have to step over some of the homeless people asleep outside. The experience truly brought the centers together. BHR and the ACI system have really come a long way. ACI was actually designed to give providers more statewide system access and reporting. The reporting requirements are quite stringent. This really strengthened the prior emergency service.

System redesign was remarkable insofar as it didn't go where it was intended to go. The work that others did brought forth some good alternatives starting at the point that we have a good system and how can we improve on it rather than overhauling it, completely redesigning it. I think for the kids, it was the start of a statewide effort to look at a system of care for kids. There was some real merit and value in bringing about change for kids.

RESPONSIBILITY FOR A SPECIFIED POPULATION: Admission criteria, service areas, target populations all applied with the broker model programs. In each case, we were responsible for a designated population.

PREVENTION AND EARLY INTERVENTION: Prevention and early intervention were never even partially realized. There is so much demand for service that you put all the resources there. There is more opportunity with the private model and there is private money. But it could be a set-aside and part of service area coordination responsibility. Funds and resources could be dedicated for prevention and early intervention in the front end of the system.

TREATING PEOPLE IN THEIR HOME COMMUNITIES: Once CPR came, I integrated it into the broker model and came up with case management teams: some intensive community support workers who did more hands-on, who made sure people got to the doctors' offices and who were out with the client as well as the broker, so that any level of care that the client needed could be managed on that team. While certain services were brokered, case management had three different levels: pure broker/wellness level, a clinical case management level and an intensive case management level. I was integrating the CPR model into the broker model because I thought that was what the broker model lacked. In fact, at Great Rivers, when I got up to a caseload of 80, I said I can't manage this population anymore. It was a resource constraint and the lack of the ability to do the intensive work, which CPR allowed to be infused. The resources that we had were the state dollars we were spending on persons who were Medicaid eligible. They could be matched, and that generated resources to fund more case managers and different levels of case management based on what the consumer needed.

CONTINUUM OF CARE: The broker model let us buy special expertise, as long as we had funds. We were not restricted to the skills of our own staff. That was the beauty of it, and it also afforded the clients choice along the continuum. They didn't have a whole lot of choice in case managers, but what they did have was a lot of choice among service providers and access to specialty providers. And geographic accessibility. That was the greatest strength of the model.

MULTIDISCIPLINARY TEAMS: Multidisciplinary teams were a challenge with the broker model because we had so many different professionals all over and the case manager was really the driver of the treatment plan and the treatment planning process in many respects. Once we were able to create more of an in-house interdisciplinary team and get in-house doctors and social workers and vocational specialists to participate in assessment and treatment plan reviews, it got strengthened. The fact that, especially with intensive treatment needs, the case manager was able to go out and meet with the client and the doctor together made all the difference in the world.

LINKAGES WITH OTHER ORGANIZATIONS: The whole model is about linkages with other organizations and agencies. Everything requires a relationship with somebody outside the system, so it became the norm rather than the exception.

FISCAL AND PROGRAMMATIC ACCOUNTABILITY: With the broker model there was a built-in case management UM/QM oversight locally, as well as the direct service. The contracting, the credentialing, the provider network management, the utilization review, the medication usage review, were all a part of that model so that we actually had providers coming in and serving on service utilization panels and reviewing other cases and we only authorized the level of service the client needed.

CITIZEN PARTICIPATION: Citizen participation came through the advisory boards, focus groups, consumer forums, outside contracted customer satisfaction and outcome measures. The advisory boards were the key to community participation. We kept the advisory boards at Great Rivers and St. Louis Mental Health and merged them. Park Hills didn't have an advisory board, so we established one. Integrated partnerships, programs and planning were a hallmark factor and the advisory boards guided all of that. That was their role.

A native of Macks Creek, Missouri, Jerry D. Osborn has drawn from the wealth of knowledge and experience he has acquired from years spent working in such diverse fields as education, finance, recreation and human services and has put them to work for mental health and substance abuse treatment services. Mr. Osborn has served as president and CEO of Pathways Community Behavioral Healthcare, Inc. since October 1987 and has led the charge to develop Pathways into the successful organization it is today. Mr. Osborn has regularly shared his knowledge, time, talents, integrity and vision through his service to professional organizations and associations in order to improve the quality and accessibility of mental health and substance abuse treatment services.

I became CEO of Community Counseling Consultants in October of 1987. At the time, we were serving clients with 18 employees out of a renovated funeral home. In the early 1990s, the board and senior management sat down and discussed where the organization was headed. I talked about my management style, my philosophy, which is the art of generally moving the herd in a westerly direction. They responded well, and what we decided was that we could not survive as a $2 million agency. So we began to add contracts. Through a combination of public and private funds, we were able to build a 24,500-square-foot facility that opened in February 1992. It houses an adolescent and adult residential treatment unit, as well as what is now our corporate, administrative offices. We had acquired several more alcohol and drug contracts, but we knew we could not survive on just those. So our idea was to look at integrating with other organizations that could benefit from participatory management.

Joe Cairns was at West Central Community Mental Health Center in Warrensburg. He and I had already talked about how we ought to put our organizations together. We were within 30 miles of each other; there would be some economies of scale. He had the clinical skills and so when Joe got his dream job of being a social worker in Kansas City, we entered into a management agreement with their board to run the organization while they decided what they wanted to do. At that point in time, Community Counseling Consultants and West Central Missouri Mental Health Center were renamed as one organization, Pathways Community Behavioral Healthcare, and its two separate governing boards merged into one.

Family Mental Health Center in Jeff City experienced a management change, and it was in fact being run by the board, and the board was having discussions about bringing others in to run the business. They called my board members and asked us to come over to talk. After the consultation, we were interested in them and their board was interested in us. They decided to integrate with us and that happened in July 1998. Their board was expanded and now serves as an advisory board that elects two members to serve on the governing board.

Also in July 1998, we bid on the state-run outpatient services contract of Southwest Missouri Mental Health Center in Nevada. We won the contract and are now providing services out of Nevada, El Dorado Springs and Butler. We added a board member from this area to the governing board to have representation from that area.

In early 1999, I received a phone call from David Duncan at Family Oriented Counseling Services (FOCUS) in Rolla. He had made some phone calls asking about our organization as they were in the process of wanting to integrate with another group. It was a good fit for both of us and they became part of Pathways in March 1999.

We have had opportunities to integrate with other organizations over the years, but we had set forth some values and principles that needed to exist before more integration would happen. One was having a contiguous landmass. I don't think you can be effective by hopscotching over great quantities of space, and our organization is already spread out enough. We have some sort of services in 31 counties. It is a long way from Belton to Farmington. It is a long way from Columbia to Nevada. I grew up in a rural area, and I know first-hand that the problem with rural areas is access. Folks don't have the means to travel very far to get service. At one point in time, we had the largest outpatient substance abuse contract in the state. We were in every little town, maybe one or two days a week, because we recognized individuals can't travel very far to get services. Our idea was to get services to as many communities as possible and replicate as nearly as you can the services offered in your larger communities. So we set about opening up a whole host of offices located throughout the service area within 30 minutes of about anywhere. In the beginning we had offices in a lot of inconvenient places that were not easily accessible. Now the offices are very much like private practitioners would have: professional buildings and offices in strip malls.

We received a telemedicine grant through the USDA in 2001 that has allowed us to really build a network among our offices. We use it for board members to be a part of the governing board meeting by video conferencing so that they do not have to make the trip to Clinton, Missouri, whenever we meet. The video conferencing allows all participants to see and talk to each other through computer screens or through TVs in the large conference rooms. It has saved us time in other areas because we have staff meetings this way as well. We are starting to have docs in say, our Rolla office, see someone in the Eldon office. It's a way to spread out our resources and bring more access to rural areas. Our psychiatrists, psychologists and nurse practitioners often travel. They go to all of our offices to see clients. They might only be there one day a week, but there is access for that one day. And so, people have access to their medications, and through their community support workers they have access anytime there would be a problem.

I've talked about contiguous areas and access, and the other important component is replication. We want to replicate, as well as we can, as many of the services that you have in the mother ship in the smallest office. And so we have done that. We are still very much a developing, evolving system because one of the things that will provide better access and better care and will be very cost effective is the use of telemedicine. We have been working to get services like this reimbursed by Medicare and Medicaid.

PREVENTION AND EARLY INTERVENTION: Another way we are involved in communities is through suicide prevention work. It is a woefully underfunded area and one that needs to be a more coordinated effort, especially with schools. By having an office location in many small towns "nearby" to almost anywhere, we have really pushed issues on suicide prevention through schools and other community organizations.

TREATING PEOPLE IN THEIR HOME COMMUNITIES: We have a program that is funded by United Way in Jeff City where we have a staff person who tries to keep at-risk individuals out of a hospital. He goes to Mid-MO and participates with discharge planning and then coordinates services for the consumers when they return home.

MULTIDISCIPLINARY TEAMS: We attempt to involve consumers in our goal of helping others. We participated when DMH trained community support assistants. They are persons with a mental illness who work with us to help their fellow consumers. We also have a thrift store that is consumer operated. We try to involve consumers in our operations; consumers participate on our Continuous Quality Improvement Committee and sit on various other committees to give us their important perspective on the things we are doing.

LINKAGES WITH OTHER ORGANIZATIONS: We encourage our local offices to be involved with other groups or organizations that are focused on mental health and substance abuse issues. Out of all of that has come our very heavy involvement with such things as federally qualified health centers. An issue that always seems to come up and one we feel like we are on the cutting edge of is diversification. We are a full-equity partner with Capital Region and St. Mary's hospitals in Jeff City; we're participating in the funding of the free clinic in Jeff City called CeMo Cares that has now taken the next step toward pursuing federally qualified status for Cole County. Pathways is also a member of CommCare.

We are involved in the communities we serve through hospitals, law enforcement, juvenile offices, Division of Family Services and others. We work very hard to make sure we are a player in the community and we do our best to embrace other players in the community. That goes for citizen participation as well. Everything from Red Ribbon campaigns to Yellow Ribbon campaigns for suicide prevention, NAMI groups and others. They all make a difference.

FISCAL AND PROGRAMMATIC ACCOUNTABILITY: As far as accountability is concerned, we go to great lengths in keeping our board very informed. I tell them I can't always bring them good news. I think that we all have to be accountable for every dollar we get and there needs to be justification for what we do with it. There is no doubt about it. But here again, I also believe that if you show me a not-for-profit that is truly not-for-profit, then I will show you one that is going out of business. We also must have dollars left, because insurance and other business costs go up every time we turn around. I want Pathways to be around to provide services to our many communities that so desperately need access to them for a long, long time.

Dorn Schuffman was appointed to direct the Missouri Department of Mental Health in December 2001. From 1996-2001 he served as director of the Division of Comprehensive Psychiatric Services.

Schuffman began his career with the department in 1978 as a planner for the Missouri Mental Health Commission. He became the department's chief of planning in 1980, coordinating the planning activities of the department's three program divisions. Schuffman was named director of Community Mental Health Services in 1984, making him responsible for the state's community mental health services budget and supervision of program certification.

He was named deputy director of Policy and Program Development in 1989. Among his responsibilities was the development of state mental health service delivery policies and procedures designed to establish and maintain a comprehensive community-based services delivery system. In 1993, Schuffman was appointed director of Heart of Missouri Mental Health Services in Columbia, a CMHC serving a ten-county area in mid-Missouri.

The relationship between DMH and the community mental health centers in Missouri is quite different than it is in many other states. It is a partnership. There are several things that have contributed to that, not the least of which was the creation of the administrative agent function during Paul Ahr's administration. But it also has to do with some of the people who have been around a long time. And I think the fact that Missouri has a commission, which gives some stability to the director's position, enables long-term relationships, trust and a partnership to develop. You have people like Kathy Carter, who has been around forever, like us, and Todd Schaible and Shirley Fearon and Bill Kyles and Karl Wilson. I think that is different from a lot of states, that there is a strong partnership between the mental health centers and the state, and that has helped both to grow. When I first started in 1979, centers were viewed as just one part of the system. Now that has changed. They *are* the system. The psychiatric facilities are related to them. It used to be that you had very separated thinking about those, and that is one of the changes that has occurred over time.

The state comprehensive mental health planning act, P.L. 99-660, really focused attention on adults with severe mental illness and children with serious emotional disturbance. That led to a change in Missouri in the populations being served and the services being provided. If you looked in the early 1980s at the services that we purchased, the primary service was psychotherapy. That was the thing that we spent the most money on. Inpatient was also up there. When you started to get more of an emphasis on persons with a serious mental illness, and kids with serious emotional disturbance, the mix of services started to change. There were some good things about that, but some things also got lost. There was more emphasis on medication services and on new services we developed like intensive case management, or what we call community support, and the CPR program, the community psychiatric rehabilitation program.

So, you had some very good things happening for adults with severe mental illness and kids with serious emotional disturbance. But the centers lost – at least through state funding and federal funding – emphasis on other populations and had to search for other funding sources to support services for people with still-serious mental health problems, but who did not fit the new state and federal target population definitions. They either had to find other funding sources or they were unable to do some of the preventive services and the school-based services that were not tied to kids with serious emotional disturbances. And so, these activities were lost in several parts of the state and I think that was an unfortunate side effect of the state comprehensive mental health planning act.

But I also think that the growth of services for adults with severe mental illness was a good thing, because it did enable us to move more and more people into community services. And when you look at the data from the early 1980s regarding who was in the hospital, and how long they stayed and whether they came back, that has changed dramatically as a result of developing more community-based services for adults with severe mental illness. The people who are in our hospitals are not the same populations that were there in the early 1980s. The emphasis at the federal level which then came down to the state level, and the growth of NAMI and their emphasis on adults with severe mental illness and MOSPAN [Missouri Statewide Parents Advisory Network] and their emphasis on children with serious emotional disturbances, had a big impact on how the centers operated in Missouri and probably all across the nation. It took a while to change over. If you look at the data, you will see that it was not until the late 1980s that you started to get a significant change.

We began getting into the Medicaid program in the late 1980s and early 1990s, and created the CPR program. It provided much more of a support to individuals so that they could remain in the community for much longer periods of time without being hospitalized. That prepared us in the early 1990s for economic hard times. John Twiehaus was the division director then. I thought at that time he did a great job with a budget problem, downsizing the hospitals significantly, being able to build replacement facilities and redirect money to the community, all at the same time. So for me, he was one of the people who did a really good job in a difficult financial situation. We redirected out of the two facilities in St. Louis and out of Farmington and out of St. Joe. In each case several million dollars got redirected from their budgets into the community services budgets. Some of that went into match for the Medicaid program that was just coming on board. And some of it went to supporting many more people in the apartment programs. If you looked at the early period of the supported community living program, the majority of people were living in residential care and skilled nursing facilities. Now, many more people are living in independent living situations, partly as a result of the redirects we were able to make out of the facilities and partly through funding from the Medicaid program.

The CPR initiative was started just prior to our budget problems. It helped when we were facing them because we had another source to grow. There was a recognition that other states were already taking advantage of a funding source that we weren't. And shortly before that, you began to have this emphasis on adults with severe mental illness and what they need, and you had the early Active Community Treatment program developing intensive case management, which we ended up calling community support, as the basis for the program.

We also had targeted case management, which came a little bit later. CPR was first; then we started to get into targeted case management, primarily for kids really. It was our experience with 503 that said this targeted case management works, and then we found out that we can bill Medicaid for it. We also had the development of all the Families First teams around the state for kids with serious emotional disturbances, and that model got added to everybody's requirements for providing services to kids. All administrative agents had to add Families First over a period of years. During that same period there was also the development of foster family homes. All of that was in the early 1990s. Also in 1990 we put into statute the ability to use non-competitive negotiation with the centers, so that was a watershed.

Splitting out Heart of Missouri and the other outpatient programs operated by the state hospitals was the initial step towards privatization. The first step was to create similar systems in all the service areas, rather than having a hospital outpatient program in one area and a mental health center in another. The idea originally was just to separate out the outpatient programs. The next step, which was a couple of years down the road, was to privatize them. The reason that privatization came about was that state operations were extremely limited in the flexibility of what they could do. The private programs that were billing Medicaid were growing rapidly and finding that they could match their dollars. The state facilities, except Great Rivers and St. Louis Mental Health Center, were stagnant. The reality was that they could have done a lot of the things that the private sector was doing, but they didn't know how. The leadership didn't have the knowledge. It was decided to privatize them, to find a private sector partner to take them over. And that proved to be a significant change for a variety of reasons, not only because those programs continued to grow and develop.

It was the same thing at the rest of the facilities: Western Missouri, Farmington and Nevada. The first step was breaking them out separately, like Great Rivers and St. Louis Mental Health Center, and then the second step was to privatize Great Rivers and St. Louis Mental Health and all the others, which resulted in their ability to attract other sources of funds and manage in a more private sector way, more flexibly. It put everybody in the same context, contrary to the early 1980s when the mental health centers were just a part of the system and the state hospitals were the other part and you had this real rivalry. And even when the state-operated outpatient providers had been split out separately, they were still state operated. There was this real "we're not all the same" competition among them. And privatizing changed the atmosphere across the state – made it a single system versus a state-operated system and a private-operated one. That was a significant change, the privatization. It was a very significant event. We were privatizing some state employees, and we had lots of concerns about their rights. Most of that went pretty well. We required the partner to employ them and keep them for a set period of time.

Also, at that same time was the creation of the crisis access system. Basically, what we did was say to the administrative agents that they needed to be responsible for 24-hour crisis response. We gave them money, but not enough money for each center to develop its whole crisis system independently. It wasn't so much intentional; we just didn't have enough money for each of them to develop their own systems. Because we only had a limited amount of money, they had to pool their resources to provide such a system. Although many centers had hotlines, what they didn't have was 24-hour face-to-face intervention. We required in the ACI that they have a multi-line phone system and that they have the ability to connect callers to a 24-hour face-to-face person, whenever it was appropriate. That was a significant change in the crisis system, and one side effect was that multiple centers had to cooperate with each other, which, I think, was one of the reasons you started to get more regional consortia of centers. In Kansas City you had the ACI and then shortly thereafter you had MC+ and managed care, which also fostered a cooperative venture. But, ACI was one of the factors that led them to pool their resources to create an organization to manage that.

I have outlined my administration with three major objectives: (1) providing leadership as the state mental health authority; (2) having integrity, that is, truly embodying the values that we espouse; and (3) stewardship, by which I mean the efficient achievement of results.

I am a strong believer that DMH is the mental health authority. But that doesn't mean that DMH does everything related to mental health. It simply means that it provides the leadership on mental health matters to Corrections, Social Services, Education and other agencies that may purchase or provide mental health services. They and other public entities like local court systems are involved with mental health. We're not going to provide all of those services or pay for everything. It is our job to provide leadership, to make sure that those services are coordinated, are of high quality and meet appropriate standards. The administrative agents – the centers – also have those responsibilities, and I think one of the challenges and opportunities that faces them is that there are a lot of other funding sources besides the DMH and they represent us in dealing with those funding sources. Just as I am responsible for working with mental health courts to promote appropriate standards of care, they need to be working with mental health courts to promote that as well at the local level, in addition to their roles as service providers.

One of the challenges that faces us all now is working with multiple providers, how to handle other providers that have an expertise and that have a capacity. That is, how to provide leadership in working with them and not try to provide the services they provide. That means working with the other alcohol and drug abuse providers who are not mental health centers. That means working with other child-serving agencies and children's residential care providers, mental health courts, mill tax boards and Division of Family Services offices. That's a big challenge for the centers: to play the local role of being the mental health leader without having to do everything. Being a leader does not mean always making the decisions; it means involving people in the appropriate way.

On the value of competence, a challenge we face is for the centers to improve their competence in a variety of ways. One of the areas is in developing integrated substance abuse and mental health treatment for persons who require that. We know it works, we know it's appropriate, and it's a matter of taking what has been our community psychiatric rehab program and integrating the appropriate substance abuse services into it and not have it an adjunct or something that you would access outside of the program. For adults with serious mental illness, a significant percentage also have a substance abuse problem. Insofar as the centers are responsible for serving persons with a serious mental illness, they have to provide substance abuse services. That doesn't mean that they serve all substance abuse clients because all substance abuse clients don't have that level of need or need the integrated services. But for those people who need that level of service, the centers have to be able to provide it.

The obverse is also true; the substance abuse providers need to have the capacity to provide the services secondary to substance abuse. So if they're dealing with somebody who is depressed because of his/her substance abuse, the agency needs to deal with the depression and not have to refer the client to deal with the depression. The same is true for persons who have a history of trauma and having an integrated program that deals with the trauma and the substance abuse or, less frequently, with trauma and mental illness. With co-occurring disorders, you have to locate the responsibility for care somewhere; it's more than coordinating services. It is going to require a significant amount of training at a time when we're having trouble recruiting and retaining training staff.

The third area is stewardship, the efficient achievement of results. That is a key one these days, and I think that is what the centers also face. For the centers it raises the question, "Who else can provide this other than us, and how do we coordinate with them, and what is underutilized?"

I think that CMHCs have a role in helping DMH fulfill its responsibilities in these areas.

6 ENDURING PRINCIPLES, EVOLVING PRIORITIES, EMERGING PRACTICES

In his history of mental health policy and practice, David Rochefort identifies a cyclical pattern of "alternating crests of high policy and program activity and troughs of stagnation and decline [89]." Proponents of this point of view are legion, and include Alexander Leighton, who commented in 1982 [68]:

> If one goes back to the origins of modern psychiatry at the close of the eighteenth century and traces what happened subsequently, it is apparent that there has been a succession of movements concerned with the care, control and prevention of mental illness. These movements have included moral treatment, mental hospital development, mental hygiene, psychoanalysis, child guidance, and, in our own time, community mental health. Each has combined very high levels of expectation with very modest levels of achievement. Thus, across almost two centuries, a wave pattern is evident: hope and activity, followed by disillusionment and turning away.

These remarks were recorded at the low point of federal support for community mental health centers, shortly after the substitution of federal block grants for the revitalizing initiatives of the Mental Health Systems Act. Recast in the light of 20 years of survival and success, they present a premature obituary for the community mental health movement, whose principles now permeate mental health service systems they once could not penetrate. As the Missouri experience teaches, long after the federal designation and funding have gone, old-line community mental health centers and their later developing cohorts perpetuate the movement because they have kept true to its principles. Forty years of experience have demonstrated that function and *philosophy*, not form, are the defining marks of a community mental health center.

RESPONSIBILITY FOR A SPECIFIED POPULATION

North Central Missouri's Executive Director Irvine [58], summarizes the ongoing importance of the service area practice, especially the CMHC's role as a safety net for persons with a mental disability:

> The principle of responsibility for a defined service area is an essential element of the CMHC system. This principle of responsibility assures that individuals within the service area will have a service provider designated to provide core services to area residents. Eliminating designated responsibility for services would make it much more likely that the neediest of the population could "fall through the cracks," as no one provider would have the designated responsibility and authority for providing services in that area.

In Missouri, this principle has been sustained in large part because DMH incorporated it as the first condition for designation of a mental health agency as an administrative agent. From the beginning of the administrative agent program, service area size was not a critical issue; in fact, when DMH reduced the number of catchment areas from 36 to 26 (and later to 25), it increased the population size of many service areas.

Furthermore, when DMH replaced the St. Louis County traveling clinic with Great Rivers Mental Health Services, it ignored the arbitrary federal formula of 75,000 to 200,000 persons per catchment area, instead creating a community mental health agency serving that county's nearly 1 million citizens, then 25% of the state's population. When St. Louis Mental Health Center was established, the outpatient programs of two former catchment areas were combined (St. Louis State Hospital and Malcolm Bliss Mental Health Center). And when Great Rivers and St. Louis Mental Health Center were privatized, BJC BH assumed responsibility for three former catchment areas, covering a population in excess of 1.2 million persons.

Similarly, in central Missouri, DMH has contracted with Pathways Behavioral Healthcare to provide comprehensive mental health services to the residents of two complete service areas and parts of two others. Economic pressures on CMHCs may foster new consolidations, and successful joint ventures like CommCare and BHR may lead to shared programs at additional service levels. Although many forces are in play to promote larger service delivery systems, Missouri's CMHC CEOs remain committed to the concept of a defined service area, and they carefully monitor the balance between service delivery efficiency and service area responsibility.

> I see a problem when service areas get too big. There are powerful and legitimate forces for consolidation, but personal knowledge of and contact with the communities we serve are absolutely vital to our success. There may be corporate structures that can address those issues and still capitalize on economies of scale, but it needs to be considered when mergers and acquisitions are proposed. [Horwitz, 53]

> I continue to believe that the service area concept is still a viable concept in the delivery of mental health services. The idea of one entity (the CMHC) having the primary responsibility for delivery of care in a geographic area assures that there is a voice for each community within the state. For certain operations, we must not think only within a service area box. CMHCs must come together in networks and resource-sharing to effectively deliver

services. This does not negate the need for planning at the service area level and the investment of the local service areas in the CMHCs. Loss of local identification and local investment will, in my belief, hasten the demise of community mental health centers. [Kyles, 66]

If the concept survives long term, I believe it will morph into a regional system of response where the most costly services, like inpatient and crisis, are shared among several service areas. This is less likely in rural areas where few providers are established. The availability of local county support is the only counter-force which may help keep the service areas distinct. Local ownership and control of CMHC programs are vital if we intend to preserve the current system. [Lebedun, 67]

PREVENTION AND EARLY INTERVENTION

The inclusion in the array of services required of a CMHC of prevention and early intervention – both hallmarks of the public health approach – was a strategy to reduce demand for services over time. Unfortunately, federal funding for these services was not available until the CMHC program was well underway. Even in Missouri, state funding for primary prevention programs was suspended in the early 1980s due to budget cuts.

Despite these obstacles, prevention and early intervention are alive and well in CMHCs throughout the state. In some cases, they are ongoing programs such as ReDiscover's *What's the Secret?* child sexual abuse prevention program that has been operating for over 15 years and is currently utilized in 68 schools. Across the state, each year Crider Center presents *Changes and Choices*, a life skills course that gets built into the school curriculum for six to twelve sessions to the majority of sixth-grade youth in its four-county service area. The program's focus is on the active training and practice of problem solving skills that can help young people avoid a variety of undesirable outcomes.

In other cases, the concepts are embodied in immediate large-scale interventions on the scene of natural and manmade disasters. On the afternoon of July 17, 1981, guests staying at the Hyatt Regency Hotel in Kansas City were mingling with local patrons as an orchestra played *Satin Doll* during an afternoon tea dance. Caught up in that festive atmosphere, hotel visitors jammed two aerial walkways overlooking the lobby. Unexpectedly, they collapsed to the floor below, trapping hundreds of other spectators and killing 111. From Western MO a few short blocks away, to the southeast and northeast reaches of Jackson County, the area's CMHCs responded at once. Immediately upon hearing of the tragedy, the DMH director contacted the governor. Within minutes, Bond directed Ahr to make $50,000 available to the Kansas City area's CMHCs as a down payment on a comprehensive crisis and follow-up response.

The readiness of CMHCs to respond immediately was no accident. Community psychiatrists, psychologists, social workers and nurses were well aware of the research of Harvard psychiatrist Dr. Erich Lindemann on the psychological aftermath of the Coconut Grove fire in Boston nearly 40 years before[60]. A dozen years later, CMHCs in eastern Missouri would step in to help their communities cope with the devastating floods that inundated the Missouri and Mississippi River region in 1993 and to aid flood victims in other states in later years. Earlier this year, CMHCs in southwest Missouri stepped in to provide crisis intervention and grief counseling to their neighbors whose property had been destroyed and whose lives had been altered by killer tornadoes.

---

[60] Near midnight on Saturday, November 28, 1942, Boston's Coconut Grove nightclub was filled beyond capacity with nearly 1,000 weekend partygoers, many of whom were preparing to go overseas on military duty. A kitchen fire spread to the ballroom, feeding on flammable ceiling and wall decorations. At the entrance, a human logjam trapped hundreds in the inferno, resulting in nearly 500 deaths. Lindemann's study [70 & 86] of the impact of this disaster on survivors and the loved ones of the victims is a classic in the field of crisis intervention.

Treating people with a mental illness in their home communities

When asked about treating people in their home communities, Lebedun [67] described what goes on at Tri-County, but he spoke for all Missouri CMHCs: "That is what we do." Although driven by an ideology that promotes treatment close to home in the least restrictive environment, Missouri CMHCs are confronted daily with a chronic shortage of available acute mental health beds. The solution to this problem sparks a lively exchange between proponents of more inpatient capacity and those promoting more community residential slots and home-based supports.

Recognizing the need for inpatient beds for persons with acute mental illnesses, Murphy [82] also commends efforts by DMH to develop non-inpatient alternatives:

> There probably never will be an alternative to inpatient treatment for those patients who become psychotically ill and require medical treatment and have a high level of safety needs. I applaud DMH for working to expand the service mix to include 24-hour emergency service with mobile outreach, crisis beds, next-day appointments and a variety of residential settings. This direction has enhanced quality by having available an appropriate service which is more cost effective and less disruptive to the patient. More such options are needed, as well as additional training to providers to assist them in using the service options.

Other commentators also point out the potential value of new alternatives to inpatient care and the benefits that can accrue from better coordination of available public and private hospital beds.

> While there is a need for 24-hour beds, that does not necessarily mean that the beds need to be in a hospital. We should work on developing small inpatient-like programs within the communities. We can take a basic residential model and beef it up with additional medical

236

services and provide an intensive level of care in small 6-to-10 bed group-home facilities in the communities at a fraction of the cost that it requires for such beds in a general hospital setting. This would also give every service area, regardless of its size and the availability of other hospitals, the capability of developing intensive 24-hour services.

The mental health industry needs to take a lesson from the substance abuse industry. Only a few years ago, there were many 30-day substance abuse inpatient facilities. Most hospitals have closed their substance abuse inpatient facilities because of poor reimbursement. The industry did not die; it retooled itself. We now have intensive residential services that take the place of what used to be very expensive inpatient services. We also have social detox and even modified medical detox being done in community settings. There is no reason that intensive psychiatric services cannot be developed in community residential settings if the proper staffing and supports are provided. [Kyles, 66]

DMH should pursue incentives to create alternatives to inpatient care. There are numerous other 24-hour options that could be created, and will likely become available, once market forces create the demand for alternatives. [Flory, 36]

Adding new beds (by construction of facilities) to the existing system of care is expensive and not generally needed. However, the integration of existing bed services on a regional basis will provide improved service to our consumers and the public. Care coordination through organizations like CommCare can link public and private bed capacity to maximize clinically correct and geographic-specific bed capacity. These systems should be supported and enhanced.

The current bed crisis has also served to revitalize the study of alternatives to hospital care such as respite or crisis beds which can be arranged through residential care facilities, hospitals, group homes and other non-traditional structures for brief overnight crisis response. [Lebedun, 67]

Wilson [110] puts the issue in a systems of care perspective:

If the bed access problem is addressed by first adding more beds, then the problem is probably never solved. All the available resources are used up in purchasing beds, and there is still a shortage. We need to develop balanced systems and focus very early on developing alternatives. This includes gaining the confidence of gatekeepers, like law enforcement, and helping them learn to use the alternative resources. We have to have a single door into hospitals, through our access systems where we have investigated every alternative. We need to find other ways of working with the courts rather than having inpatient facilities be the dumping grounds for forensic patients. Many forensic patients are very high functioning and do not need to use up a psychiatric inpatient bed resource.

CONTINUUM OF CARE

While the principle of a continuum of care has remained constant since the earliest days of the CMHC movement, the components of the continuum periodically have changed. The first federally funded CMHCs were required to offer 5, then 12, services; that list was changed again under the ADAMH block grants. In the mid 1960s, the Executive Committee for Mental Health Planning [30] described ten services Missouri's three proposed regional intensive treatment centers would be expected to provide. Service system reforms in Missouri in the early 1980s established three levels of service continua for its administrative agents: core and intermediate clinics and full service centers. A decade later, a new CPR continuum was introduced, as were comprehensive approaches to services for children with serious emotional disorders. As recently as 1999, the Federation of Missouri Advocates detailed the elements of a comprehensive system of care in its response to DMH's proposed system redesign initiative [31].

At the present time, the robustness of a CMHC's continuum of care is marked by two elements. At the base, CMHCs are providing the set of services required by DMH to meet the needs of some consumers in the department's target groups. At the high end, CMHCs continue to provide a full range of services for adults with a serious mental illness and children and youth with a serious emotional disturbance, as well as some of the more traditional prevention, early intervention and mental health counseling services for persons not counted among the DMH target groups.

The factors that contribute to the variability in service offerings are multiple. They include the state's increasing reliance on Medicaid as a funding source, the requirements of other funding sources, the concentration of persons with a serious mental illness/emotional disturbance in a service area, the availability of other mental health agencies and providers within the service area, as well as the availability of trained staff to implement programs and services.

These conditions notwithstanding, the bottom line for many Missouri CMHCs is that in the years since 1981, DMH's share of state general revenue dollars has eroded from more than 10% of the state general fund to less than 6.5% [54]. Even during the prosperous 1990s, DMH service providers were routinely bypassed when cost-of-living and other rate adjustments were distributed to other human service and education entities. Funding for DMH clients has not kept pace with demand or with the cost to provide these services in the private sector [5]. Failure to restore funding for DMH provider agencies will contribute to the further constriction of service choices for Missourians who need mental health care.

One area of potential relief lies in the passage of county mill taxes to support a balanced program of community mental health services. In the area of developmental disabilities, more than 80 of the 114 Missouri counties and the City of St. Louis have passed such taxes. In the mental health arena, only one dozen have done so. The challenge is impressive, and the roles are clear. Interested citizens must be mobilized to defend and expand the services provided by their local CMHCs. Local initiatives will benefit from a strict application of former Missouri Attorney General Ashcroft's opinion on the distribution of mill tax monies.

In the 1990s, public mental health programs in Missouri were sustained by an aggressive push to enroll consumers in Medicaid-funded services. This strategy provided funding, but at a stiff price: the near conversion of CMHC caseloads to financially and medically eligible Medicaid clients. In this decade, an equally aggressive push to pass local mental health taxes will help reverse that trend by making funds available – once again – for a full continuum of care that is affordable, accessible and appropriate to the needs of *all* Missourians.

MULTIDISCIPLINARY TEAMS

From the earliest days of public mental hospitals, through the era of mental hygiene and child guidance clinics, the mental health field has enjoyed a long history of team-based treatment. This tradition remains a key component of CMHC care today. The early 1970s saw an interest in employing in a paraprofessional role former recipients of mental health services and other community members, who supplemented a professional staff replete with psychiatrists, clinical psychologists, clinical social workers and psychiatric nurses. When economic hard times hit, many of these positions were eliminated to conserve resources to pay the salaries of the professional staff. Today, CMHCs in Missouri use paraprofessional staff to an extent that far exceeds the earlier practice. Consumers of mental health services, parents of children with serious emotional disorders, and other clients fill important roles as in crisis intervention and wraparound services. Efforts to employ community members as CMHC staff provided an important opportunity for many – especially persons living in economically distressed communities.

In recent years, research on the effects of cultural competence on treatment outcomes in mental health care[61] has raised the issue of multicultural teams to a high level of importance. Two CMHC CEOs from Missouri's urban settings have addressed this issue. For Jackson County's Kyles [66],

> There is an increasing disconnect between the cultural and ethnic makeup of providers and that of consumers in the public sector. Minorities, like the rest of the general population, are not being attracted to the psychiatric service professions. This must be turned around. There is an increasing need for cultural diversity and cultural competency within mental health programs. Unfortunately, due to a variety of factors, the move to make programs culturally competent is not gaining great momentum. This is partially due to budgetary concerns, lack of appropriate staffing and lack of commitment by mental health authorities. This will only be turned around when mental health authorities require cultural competency as one of the basic measures of the ability of mental health programs to receive funding.

> The mental health community has to address the cultural diversity crisis in staffing as a whole. The community must come up with ways to provide public education to persuade minorities to go into the mental health professions, to increase salaries in the mental health professions and to increase realistic opportunities for advancement within the mental health professions. We must start at the high school level convincing young people that a career in mental health is rewarding. We must have mentoring programs that will allow for the professional development of paraprofessional minorities. In Missouri, both DMH and the Coalition have formed committees and task forces to

---

[61] See Ahr [5] Issue #7: *Cultural Proficiency.*

come up with solutions. Time will tell how successful we will be.

St. Louis' Murphy [82] suggests that cultural diversity efforts

...should not focus on any one group. Programs popping up to address the so-called "new American" as an example, can lead to resentment, since the issue of the "old American" has not been adequately addressed. Thus, it would be wise to have broad-based programs with intense training to change attitudes and increase knowledge on diversity so that the diverse needs of many groups can be met. One approach would be to identify and focus on key areas that apply to any racial, ethnic, or cultural group, for example: respect, ability to communicate with the group, knowledge of the group culture, knowledge of research on the group such as members' reactions to drugs and openness to accepting service.

Direct services best serve patients when they are available close to the natural environment and are easy to access and culturally competent, which is sometimes best achieved by employing persons from the natural environment.

Finally, Lebedun [67] points out that an outsourcing strategy can address both issues.

A contract with a private provider can be negotiated to provide specialized service to virtually any consumer needing it. Diversity (religious, racial, gender, etc.) can be addressed by locating providers who fit the profile of consumers needing care. This matching ability is possible most easily in a networked system. It also allows shared staffing between like-minded agencies.

LINKAGES WITH OTHER ORGANIZATIONS

CMHCs were always expected to work closely with other human service agencies in their communities. In fact, the intent of mandated consultation services was to improve the mental health case finding and intervention skills of practitioners in such agencies. The practice of linkage has grown, especially as human service agencies have proliferated and as scarce resources have become scarcer. Some agencies, such as Great Rivers Mental Health Services in St. Louis County and Tri-County Mental Health Services in Kansas City, were designed to directly access and pay for services from other community practitioners and agencies. The emergence of consumer and family-of-consumer organizations has provided an additional opportunity for CMHC linkages.

Over the past six years, CMHCs have entered into formal linkages with each other to form larger, regional service units. Two examples of this activity are the establishment of regional joint ventures such as CommCare in western Missouri and BHR in the east and the consolidation of several smaller mental health agencies into Pathways Behavioral Healthcare. For some observers of Missouri's CMHC system, further economic pressure, especially from state sources, may trigger further consolidations of smaller CMHCs into larger mental health or health systems of care.

For many in the field of community mental health, linking with a local health care system is a logical arrangement[62]. However, in Missouri, such affiliations have not been universally sustainable. The first three federally funded CMHCs, although freestanding entities, were co-located with general hospitals at major medical center sites. With privatization, the outpatient programs of these

---

[62] Commenting on the first ten years of the CMHC program, Dr. Jack Ewalt [29], former Joint Commission director, spoke directly to the issue of CMHCs being a part of hospital systems:

The community mental health centers, as finally developed by [NIMH], were somewhat different from what we [the Joint Commission members] had originally planned. Our view had been that we should go from a psychiatric base in medicine in the community, much in the manner of the old travelling clinics, and that the home base would be the local hospital with a psychiatric unit...I believe the [NIMH] modification to make the programs still more comprehensive was probably a good one. Our recommendation that the clinic should be fitted to the needs and resources of the community was implemented. I still think our recommendations for community clinics were sound.

three CMHCs were incorporated into large health systems (Mid-MO to the University of Missouri Health Care, Western MO to Truman and the St. Louis and Farmington area programs to BJC HealthCare).

Of the remaining 13 federal CMHC grant recipients, eight were hospitals or comprehensive health centers. Two hospital-based grantees withdrew from the program at an early stage. Only one of the remaining six grantees which developed mature CMHC operations, Swope Health Services, continues to operate a CMHC. One CMHC that had been federally funded was incorporated into a health system in 1984 and was recently spun off, after 19 years. Two other CMHCs that had been federally funded were subsequently incorporated into regional health systems. No private CMHC that had not been a federal CMHC grantee has become a part of a health system.

Observations by current Missouri CMHC chiefs reflect the alternate points of view that surround this issue. Family Guidance's Hammond [49] has developed a convenient summary of the main advantages and disadvantages of linkage with a health system, to which the commentaries of other CMHC CEOs have been added.

Advantage #1: Better integration with primary care.

> This would allow CMHCs to more easily access and treat individuals (assuming they have a payor source) who are not in DMH's target populations. There are known advantages to integrating behavioral health into primary care. Certainly, consolidating a CMHC with a hospital/ health system may allow this to occur more easily and efficiently. [Hammond, 49]

> Linkage with a health system can provide an important conduit for CMHCs to reach patients who need integrated care services. Many chronic diseases like diabetes and hypertension have improved treatment outcomes when mental health care is part of the intervention. Similarly,

many mental health patients have serious health problems that must be addressed if their overall condition is to improve. Linkage in this context is not taken to mean a structural merger with a hospital. [Lebedun, 67]

Major advantages of consolidating CMHC operations into large health systems include clients being able to get holistic health and mental health care readily accessible and integrated. Clients should experience increased benefits in both health and mental health areas. Negative drug interaction side effects should be reduced. Taking better care of the clients' physical health side should help improve their mental health and vice versa. [Kyles, 66]

If the organization is correctly structured, there is an increased opportunity to coordinate care between mental health and physical health care. The primary care physician and the psychiatrist can co-locate, communicate and learn from each other. There is an increased possibility for a comprehensive medication profile, complete assessment and improved client satisfaction. [Morgan, 80]

Short of consolidation, there continually needs to be better coordination among substance abuse, mental health and primary health care. Changes need to be made in the Medicaid and Medicare system of paying to help encourage treating the whole person. [Steinmetz, 99]

Advantage #2: Possible reduced administrative costs through economies of scale.

Some areas of potential strengths are in shared administrative functions, thus saving resources. Clinical areas for potential sharing include emergency services, discharge planning and inpatient psychiatric consultations. Work with primary care physicians is also highly desirable, especially in high-volume offices or with large Medicaid populations. [Flory, 36]

Many hospitals have more extensive resources than do CMHCs. These resources provide infrastructure to all programs. Hospitals also have opportunities to bill a variety of sources and can incorporate mental health services into contracts, thereby enhancing the payer portfolio. There are several areas where hospitals can provide support. The increasing level of compliance adds overhead disproportionately to smaller organizations. Consolidation helps disperse the costs of increasing regulations. Other departments, such as public relations, human resources and information technology, can provide support to the CMHC at a level that is not easily affordable by the CMHC alone. [Morgan, 80]

One of the main advantages to this linkage is the availability of the health system's infrastructure capacities to the community mental health center's operations. These can include information management systems, quality management programs and techniques, risk management, human resources, and perhaps most important, cash flow. The community mental health center can achieve economies of scale by utilizing these infrastructure systems of a larger health care system. [Stansberry, 97]

Advantage #3: Access to charitable dollars through hospital/health system development office efforts.

Non-profit hospitals/health systems typically have large, well-staffed development offices. This allows the corporation to have a range of development initiatives. Directing some of the development projects and monies to the CMHC could allow the CMHC to be less dependent on government funding. Voluntary dollars could strengthen under-funded programs and could be used to educate the public about mental illness. [Hammond, 49]

Disadvantage #1: Loss of core mission.

CMHCs pride themselves on reaching out to those with the most severe mental health needs. This mission or focus may not be shared by the hospital/health system. Programs and services for DMH's target population are underfunded and heavily regulated. Further, some populations served by CMHCs, such as forensic and Department of Corrections clients, generate little or no public support. [Hammond, 49]

Community mental health isn't well understood by large health systems and it is a very small part of a medical and surgical hospital enterprise. Consequently, it is sometimes difficult to get the support and attention we need to develop. These systems also tend to think in terms of integration into the larger system – how can behavioral health support general health care? While this is an exciting direction for community mental health to grow, services for persons with a serious and persistent mental illness aren't such a good fit. [Horwitz, 53]

Our role as a community mental health center is greater than service delivery; it encompasses training, community education and advocacy responsibilities. These may not be consistent with the mission of any particular health system. [Huss, 56]

One of the major disadvantages of the health system/ mental health linkage is that the community mental health center can be an outlier within the health system. Most health systems are comprised of large medical/surgical hospitals, and the operation of a community mental health center is relatively small (in terms of finances and statistics) when it is compared to the operation of the hospital(s). This can lead to the problem of the community mental health center being placed in the position of being misunderstood within the context of its service delivery system. [Stansberry, 97]

Disadvantage #2: Restriction of treatment models.

CMHCs must take a pragmatic approach to developing programs to meet the needs of those they serve. No one treatment model fits all needs. Integration with primary care is appropriate for some individuals. However, others would advocate that CMHCs are a blend of medical and social service models. A hospital/health system may not be comfortable with a CMHC that doesn't fit into a medical model. [Hammond, 49]

Disadvantage #3: Increased costs.

It is conceivable that consolidating a CMHC into a hospital/health system would increase the expense of operation for the CMHC by how overhead expenses are allocated. Administrative, accreditation, building and other expenses might be assigned to the CMHC, creating increased fiscal pressure on the CMHC. [Hammond, 49]

Large hospital systems often do not provide a strong support system for mental health. In fact, they may degrade resources away from outpatient and prevention services that are vital for a community approach. [Lebedun, 67]

The extent to which a CMHC partners with a hospital/health system will ultimately depend on local conditions. The extent to which a CMHC *successfully* partners with a hospital/health system will depend on factors such as compatibility of mission, values and prime service areas, as well as a shared commitment to serving consumers with a limited ability to pay for their care.

Whether a hospital/health system and a CMHC should consolidate can only be answered by the local entities carefully evaluating the advantages and disadvantages mentioned plus many more. Compatibility of community need, corporate culture, mission and strategic vision all need to be reviewed and debated before a consolidation decision could be reached. [Hammond, 49]

While there are advantages to consolidating CMHC operations into larger health systems, I believe that moving in this direction requires the following:

- There must be some compelling reason to consolidate other than finances.
- The two parts must have common features in order to create a strong and long-lasting bond. Examples include common/similar mission, common population, shared geography.
- The two parts should have complementary strengths.
- The organization must be carefully structured so that mental health has a presence at the executive level.
- Hospital leaders must be willing to learn about mental health services, as this product line is substantially different from any other line of business. [Morgan, 80]

FISCAL AND PROGRAMMATIC ACCOUNTABILITY

In the beginning, federal funding for CMHC services was in the form of multi-year grants. Proposals were filed with DHEW, budgets were reviewed, grants were made and reports were required to justify further Congressional appropriations. Failure to perform in a specific area typically merited technical assistance from "the feds," and the proposal, review, budget, allocation and documentation process began again. As their federal funding began to wane, Missouri's CMHCs promoted a fee-for-service reimbursement arrangement with DMH. This funding mechanism was at the opposite end of the reimbursement continuum from multi-year guaranteed grants. This approach has dominated DMH-CMHC fiscal accountability arrangements ever since. Whenever centers secure other public or private funding, these funding sources impose their own typically unique financial and reporting requirements. With multiple funding sources comes multiple reporting requirements.

CITIZEN PARTICIPATION:

Citizen participation in governance has continued as a hallmark of CMHCs in Missouri. Although they were not at first required by NIMH, eventually all federally funded centers established boards of directors that included representatives of community and professional stakeholder groups. DMH reinforced this concept when it established the administrative agent system. Even where Missouri's CMHCs were incorporated into larger organizations, the expectation of a broadly representative governing or advisory board has been maintained. Over time, CMHCs have supplemented these early forms of citizen participation with a variety of advisory councils and focus groups and through consumer satisfaction research. Perhaps, the greatest boost to high-quality citizen participation, however, has been the steadfast advocacy of the MHA and the emergent relevance over the past two decades of other powerful advocacy groups, especially NAMI and MOSPAN.

EPILOGUE

Late in William Hanley's play about Mrs. Dally [50], his heroine and her young friend Frankie quietly discuss the nature of their relationship. Reflecting on his promise to one day reciprocate her kindness to him, Mrs. Dally gently suggests that later on someone else will get back from Frankie all that she had given to him:

> MRS. DALLY: It's like that game we used to play when I was a kid: Pass It On. You ever play that? You'd say something to the kid next to you, or do something and tell him to pass it on. Sometimes it was something nice, sometimes it was a punch in the arm. Being alive is a lot like that game.

Being committed to the principles of community mental health is a lot like that game, also. Most of the time, it feels nice; sometimes it feels like a punch in the arm. Above all else, it makes you feel alive. In the last 40 years, we who once were like Frankie: naïve, uncertain, idealistic, are now more like Mrs. Dally: aware of the positive impact we have had on the lives of others, grateful for the opportunity to participate in this grand and successful venture, eager to enroll others in its important mission. Much has changed; our dedication to serving our neighbors with a mental illness or emotional disturbance in and near their homes and places of play, work and worship has remained the same. Acknowledging those who came before, we best can echo Mrs. Dally when we gently suggest to those who come next: PASS IT ON.

REFERENCES

1. Advisory Commission on Intergovernmental Relations. 1977. *Block Grants: A Comparative Analysis.* Washington, D.C.: U.S. Government Printing Office.

2. Ahr, P.R. 1980. *Creating a partnership: State, local and federal responsibilities for the mentally ill.* Unpublished manuscript. Jefferson City, MO: Missouri Department of Mental Health.

3. Ahr, P.R. 1981. Proposals to reduce the DMH budget for FY 1981 by $18,717,449: A report to the Missouri Mental Health Commission, January 17, 1981. Unpublished manuscript. Jefferson City, MO: Missouri Department of Mental Health.

4. Ahr P.R. 1991. Administering state mental health programs: The evolution of the contemporary state agency. In C. G. Cox and A. J. Hudson (Eds.), *Dimensions of State Mental Health Policy.* New York: Praeger.

5. Ahr, P.R. 2002. *Notes for the Vigilant, the Active, the Brave: Certain issues for uncertain times.* St. Louis: Causeway.

6.   Ashcroft, J.D. 1981. Attorney General Opinion No. 31. Jefferson City, MO: Office of the Attorney General of Missouri.

7.   Beers, C.W. 1913. *A Mind that Found Itself.* New York, Longmans, Green & Co.

8.   Binner, P., Evenson, R. and Evenson, J. 1994. *The 503 Project: Performance and evaluation report.* St. Louis: Missouri Institute of Mental Health.

9.   Bockoven, J. S. 1963. *Moral Treatment in American Psychiatry.* New York: Springer.

10.   Brand, J. L. 1965. The National Mental Health Act of 1946: A retrospective. *Bulletin of the History of Medicine,* 39: 231-245.

11.   Brand, J.L. 1967. *The United States: An historical perspective.* In R. H. Williams & L. D. Ozarin, *Community Mental Health: An International Perspective.* San Francisco: Jossey-Bass.

12.   Caplan, G. 1956. Mental health consultation in schools. In: *The Elements of a Community Mental Health Program.* New York: Millbank Memorial Fund.

13.   Caplan, G. 1963. Types of mental health consultation. *American Journal of Orthopsychiatry,* 33: 470-481.

14.   Caplan, G. 1964. *Principles of Preventive Psychiatry.* New York: Basic Books.

15.   Caplan, G. 1970. *The Theory and Practice of Mental Health Consultation.* New York: Basic Books.

16.   Chang, C.F., Kiser, L.J., Bailey, J.E., Martins, M., Gibson, W.C., Schaberg, K.A., Mirvis, D.M. & Applegate, W.B. 1998. Tennessee's failed managed care program for mental

health and substance abuse services. *Journal of the American Medical Association,* 279: 864-869.

17. Compton, F. 2003. Personal communication.

18. Congressional Record: July 24, 1980, pp. 9720-9743.

19. Congressional Record: August 22, 1980, pp. H7601-H7607.

20. Cravens, R.B. 1981. Grassroots participation in community mental health. In W. H. Silverman (Ed.), *Community Mental Health: A sourcebook for professionals and advisory board members.* New York: Praeger.

21. Cravens, R.B. 2003. Personal communication.

22. Crighton, J.C. 1993. *The History of Health Services in Missouri.* Omaha, NE: Barnhart Press.

23. Cumming, E. and Cumming, J. 1957. *Closed Ranks: An Experiment in Mental Health Education.* Cambridge, MA: Harvard University Press.

24. Davidson, H.A. 1953. Psychiatry and the euphemistic delusion. *The American Journal of Psychiatry* 110: 311-312.

25. Deutsch, A. 1948. *The Shame of the States.* New York: Harcourt, Brace and Co.

26. Deutsch, A. 1949. *The Mentally Ill in America.* 2nd ed. New York: Columbia University Press.

27. Dickens, C. 1842. *American Notes for General Circulation* (Vol. 1). London: Chapman & Hall.

28. Evans, T. St. Louis *American.* Elders keynotes health care salute. May 22-28, 2003.

29.   Ewalt, J. 1975. The birth of the community mental health movement. In W.E. Barton and C. J. Sanborn (Eds.) *An Assessment of the Community Mental Health Movement.* Lexington, MA: Lexington Books.

30.   Executive Committee for Comprehensive Mental Health Planning. 1966. *Comprehensive Mental Health Planning in Missouri.* Columbia, MO: The University of Missouri School of Medicine.

31.   Federation of Missouri Advocates for Mental Health and Substance Abuse Services. 1999. *Reasonable Expectations for the Design and Operation of a System of Publicly Funded Psychiatric and Substance Abuse Treatment Services and Supports: A Public Response to the Missouri Department of Mental Health's Paper: Implementing Missouri's "Show Me System Redesign."* Jefferson City: Federation of Missouri Advocates for Mental Health and Substance Abuse Services.

32.   Felix, R. H. 1963. Comments: Community mental health centers. *The American Journal of Psychiatry,* 120: 506-507.

33.   Felix, R. H. 1964. Community mental health: A federal perspective. *The American Journal of Psychiatry,* 121: 428-432.

34.   Felix, R. H. 1967. *Mental Illness: Progress and Prospects.* New York: Columbia University Press.

35.   Felix, R. H. 1971. The challenges – past, present and future. Reprinted in *Mental Health Challenges: Past and Future: Proceedings of a conference on the twenty-fifth fifth anniversary of the National Mental Health Act.* Rockville, MD: National Institute of Mental Health.

36.   Flory, A. 2003. Personal communication.

37. Foley, H. 1975. *Community Mental Health Legislation: The Formative Process.* Lexington, MA: D.C. Heath and Company, Lexington Books.

38. Frazier, C. Testimony before the Committee on Foreign and Interstate Commerce. U.S. Congress, House, 1963: 350.

39. Fujita, M.T. 2003. Personal communication.

40. Goffman, E. 1961. *Asylums: Essays on the Social Situation of Mental Patients and Other Inmates.* Garden City, NY: Doubleday, Anchor Books.

41. Golann, S.E. and Eisdorfer, C. 1972. Mental health and the community: The development of issues. In S.E. Golann and C. Eisdorfer (Eds.) *Handbook of Community Mental Health.* New York: Appleton-Century-Crofts.

42. Goode, E. 2003. Leading drugs for psychosis come under new scrutiny. New York *Times.* May 20, 2003.

43. Goodwin, C. 1965. Troubled find help at unique Ozark Psychiatric Foundation in Joplin. The Joplin *Globe*, February 12, 1965.

44. Grob, G.N. 1991. *From Asylum to Community: Mental Health Policy in Modern America.* Princeton: Princeton University Press.

45. Guhleman, H.V. 2000. Henry V. Guhleman, M.D.: Pioneering the state mental health system. *The Mental Health Reporter*, XV, (12), 20-21.

46. Guhleman, H.V. 2001. Governor's suicide calls attention to mental illness. *The Mental Health Reporter,* XV1, (1), 8-9.

47. Guhleman, H.V. 2001. The mental health crisis of 1961. *The Mental Health Reporter,* XV1, (2), 10-13.

48. Guhleman, H.V. 2003. Personal communication.

49. Hammond, G. 2003. Personal communication.

50. Hanley, W. 1965. Mrs. Dally has a lover. In E. Parone (Ed.) *New Theatre in America*. New York: Dell.

51. Hargreaves, W.A., Attkisson, C.C., Siegel, L.M., McIntyre, M.H. and Sorensen, J.E. (Eds.) 1974. *Resource materials for community mental health program evaluation*. San Francisco: National Institute of Mental Health.

52. Holahan, J., Zuckerman, S., Evans, A. & Rangarajan, S. 1988. Medicaid managed care in thirteen states. *Health Affairs*, 17: 43-63.

53. Horwitz, B. 2003. Personal communication.

54. House, J.E. 2003. Personal communication.

55. Hurley, R.E .& Draper, D.A. 1998. Medicaid managed care for special populations: Behavioral health as a "tracer condition." *New Directions in Mental Health Services*, 78: 51-65.

56. Huss, S. 2003, Personal communication.

57. Hyde, P.S. 1996. Creating incentives for the delivery of services. *New Directions in Mental Health Sservices*. 72: 25-34.

58. Irvine, L. 2003. Personal communication.

59. Jerrell, J.M. and Larsen, J.K. 1984. Policy shifts and organizational adaptation: A review of current developments. *Community Mental Health Journal* 20: 282-293.

60. Jerrell, J.M. and Larsen, J.K. 1985. How community mental health centers deal with cutbacks and competition.

Hospital and Community Psychiatry, 36: 1169-1174.

61. Jerrell, J.M. and Larsen, J.K. 1986. Community mental health services in transition: Who is benefiting? *American Journal of Orthopsychiatry,* 56: 78-88.

62. Joint Commission of Mental Illness and Health 1961. *Action for Mental Health.* New York: Basic Books.

63. Jones, M. 1968. *Social Psychiatry in Practice: The Idea of a Therapeutic Community.* New York: Penguin.

64. Kennedy, J.F. 1963. *Message of the President of the United States Relative to Mental Illness and Mental Retardation.* 88th Congress, First Session, U.S. House of Representatives Document No. 58. U.S. Government Printing Office.

65. Kirven, L.E., Jr. 1976. Personal communication.

66. Kyles, W. 2003. Personal communication.

67. Lebedun, M. 2003. Personal communication.

68. Leighton, A.H. 1982. *Caring for Mentally Ill People: Psychological and Social Barriers in Historical Context.* Cambridge: Cambridge University Press.

69. Lille-Blanton, M. & Lyons, B. 1998. Managed care and low-income populations: recent state experiences. *Health Affairs,* 17: 238-247.

70. Lindemann, E. 1944. Symptomatology and management of acute grief. *American Journal of Psychiatry,* 101: 141-148.

71. Mannio, F.V., MacLennan, B.W. and Shore, M.F. 1975. *The Practice of Mental Health Consultation.* New York: Gardner.

72. McFarland, D. 2003. Personal communication.

73. Mechanic, D. 1998. The changing face of mental health managed care. *New Directions in Mental Health Services,* 78: 7-13.

74. Mechanic, D., Schlesinger, M. & McAlpine, D.D. 1995. Management of mental health and substance abuse services: state of the art and early results. *Millbank Quarterly,* 73: 15-53.

75. Missouri Department of Mental Health 1981. Minutes of the December 1981 meeting of the Missouri Mental Health Commission. Jefferson City, MO: Missouri Department of Mental Health.

76. Missouri Department of Mental Health 1981. *Consolidated Plan Update Fiscal Years 1982-1984.* Jefferson City, MO: Missouri Department of Mental Health.

77. Missouri Department of Mental Health 1991. *Implementing Missouri's "Show Me System Redesign".* Jefferson City, MO: Missouri Department of Mental Health.

78. Missouri General Assembly, Committee on Legislative Research 1947. *The Mentally Ill.* Jefferson City, MO.

79. Missouri State Auditor. 2003. Division of Comprehensive Psychiatric Services Contracts for Services (Audit Number 2003-86). Jefferson City, MO.

80. Morgan, M. 2003. Personal communication.

81. Moynihan, D.P. 1969. *Maximum Feasible Misunderstand--ing.* New York: Free Press.

82. Murphy, A. 2003. Personal communication.

83. Naierman, N., Haskins, B. and Robinson, G. 1978. *Community Mental Health Centers – A Decade Later.* Cambridge, MA: Abt Books.

84. National Institute of Mental Health 1971. *Community Mental Health Centers Program Operating Handbook Part I: Policy and standards manual.* Washington, D.C.: Department of Health, Education and Welfare Public Health Service.

85. Nutting, J. 1902. The poor, the defective and the criminal. In E. Fields (Ed.) *State of Rhode Island and Providence Plantations at the End of the Century.* Boston: Mason.

86. Parad, H. 1965. *Crisis Intervention: Selected readings.* New York: Family Service Association of America.

87. Ray, C.G. 2003. Personal communication.

88. Register, D. 1974. Community mental health – For whose community? *American Journal of Public Health,* 64: 886-893.

89. Rochefort, D. A. 1997. *From Poorhouses to Homelessness: Policy Analysis and Mental Health Care.* 2nd ed. Westport, CT: Auburn House.

90. Roebuck, L.B. 2003. Personal communication.

91. Rothbard, A. 1999. Managed mental health care for seriously mentally ill populations. *Current Opinion in Psychiatry*, 12: 211-216.

92. St. Louis *Missouri Republican*, July 17, 1870, 4.

93. Schnibbe, H.C. 1981. Personal communication.

94. Schulberg, H.C., Sheldon, A. and Baker, F. 1969. *Program Evaluation in the Health Fields.* New York: Behavioral Publications.

95. Singh, R.K.J. 1971. *Community Mental Health Consultation and Crisis Intervention.* Berkeley, CA: Book People.

96. Spokane system redesign brings decline in rehab services. *Mental Health Weekly* 1999: Vol. 9, No.29, pp. 1, 4.

97. Stansberry, M. 2003. Personal communication.

98. Stanton, A.H. and Schwartz, M.H. 1954. *The Mental Hospital: A Study of Institutional Participation in Psychiatric Illness and Treatment.* New York: Basic Books.

99. Steinmetz, R. 2003. Personal communication.

100. Stuart, M & Weinrich, M. 1998. Beyond managing Medicaid costs: restructuring care. *Millbank Quarterly,* 76: 251-280.

101. Swan, B. 1946. Roger Williams and the Insane. *Rhode Island History,* 5: 65-70.

102. Szasz, T. 1961. *The Myth of Mental Illness.* New York: Harper and Row.

103. Tice, N.J. 2003. Personal communication.

104. Ulett, G.A. 1962. The Bliss story: Impact of research programs upon a public mental hospital. *Psychiatric Research Reports*, 15, 29-31.

105. Ulett, G.A. 1970. Ten years of mental health progress in Missouri – Next step? *Missouri Medicine*, 772-782, 823-824.

106. Ulett, G.A. 1989. Commentaries: History of the Division of Mental Diseases: Part II, Directorships of Drs. Duval and Ulett. *Missouri Psychiatry*, 18 (1), 13.

107. Ulett, G.A. 1989. Commentaries: History of the Division of Mental Diseases: Part III, The Establishment of the Missouri Institute of Psychiatry. *Missouri Psychiatry*, 18 (2), 25.

108.   Virginia Legislative Audit and Review Commission 1979. *Deinstitutionalization and community services.* Richmond, VA.

109.   Ward, M.J. 1946. *The Snake Pit.* New York: Random House.

110.   Wilson, K. 2003. Personal communication.

111.   Zusman, J. 1975. The philosophic basis for community and social psychiatry. In W.E. Barton and C.J. Sanborn (Eds.) *An Assessment of the Community Mental Health Movement.* Lexington, MA: Lexington Books.

112.   Zusman, J. and Wurster, C.R. 1975. *Program Evaluation: Alcohol, Drug Abuse and Mental Health Services.* Lexington, MA: Lexington Books.

ABOUT THE AUTHOR

Since 1968, Dr. Paul R. Ahr has functioned in a variety of roles in the field of mental health: practicing clinician, public administrator and national mental health consultant. He was awarded the Doctor of Philosophy degree in Clinical Psychology by the Catholic University of America and the Master of Public Administration degree by the University of Southern California. While Chief Psychologist at the U.S. Naval Hospital in Oakland, California, Dr. Ahr began his post-doctoral studies in community mental health at the Center for Training in Community Psychiatry and Mental Health Administration at Berkeley, California. In 1972, he was awarded a NIMH Post-Doctoral Fellowship to study at the Laboratory of Community Psychiatry at the Harvard Medical School in Boston, Massachusetts.

In 1973, Dr. Ahr was named the first director of children's programs for the Virginia Department of Mental Health and Mental Retardation in Richmond. By 1975, he was appointed assistant commissioner for the Virginia department. He also was a consultant to the federal Department of Health, Education and Welfare (DHEW) on CMHC grants and operations. Dr. Ahr served as a consultant to the President's Commission on Mental Health and participated in the writing of its final report. He also spearheaded the drafting of the proposed Partnership for Mental Health Act of 1979, NASMHPD's comprehensive response to early DHEW drafted Mental Health Systems Act legislation.

From 1979 to 1986, Dr. Ahr was director of the Missouri Department of Mental Health in Jefferson City. As director, he worked with the Missouri General Assembly to modernize state mental health statutes, and streamlined and strengthened linkages between the department and its community mental health provider network. While in that post he was elected NASMHPD president.

In 1986, Dr. Ahr established The Altenahr Group, Ltd., which now serves an international client base from its offices in St. Louis, Missouri and Miami Beach, Florida. From 1986 to 2002, Dr. Ahr concurrently served as National Mental Health Advisor for Ernst & Young, LLP. In that capacity, he consulted with state mental health departments and community mental health programs in 25 states. In addition, he collaborated with the Missouri Coalition of Community Mental Health Centers and other mental health interest groups in Missouri to successfully counter state proposals to convert the Missouri mental health system to a for-profit managed care approach. In 2001, he was awarded the *Silver Key Award* by the Mental Health Association of Greater St. Louis in recognition of his on-going dedication to improving the care and treatment of persons with a mental illness or serious emotional disturbance.

Dr. Ahr has taught mental health, health and public administration and psychology as a member of the faculties of Boston University, the University of Southern California, Virginia Commonwealth University and its Medical College of Virginia. He is currently on the teaching faculty in the graduate Department of Health Management and Informatics of the University of Missouri-Columbia.

Dr. Paul R. Ahr is the author of *Notes for the Vigilant, the Active, the Brave: Certain issues for uncertain times* (St. Louis: Causeway, 2002), 18 observations on the challenges facing the Missouri Department of Mental Health and its provider networks at the beginning of the 21st century. He also co-authored *Overturn Turnover: Why some employees leave, why some employees stay, and ways to keep the ones who you want to stay* (St. Louis: Causeway, 2000) with Dr. Thomas B. Ahr.

NAMES INDEX

SUBJECT INDEX

National Association of State Mental Health Program Directors (NASMHPD), 48, 56, 188, 265-266.

National Committee for Mental Hygiene, 27, 32

National Council for Community Behavioral Healthcare, 10, 91, 161

National Institute of Mental Health, 28-29, 31, 36, 39, 41, 44-45, 48-49, 52, 56-57, 71, 74-75, 81, 105-106, 143, 243, 250, 265,

National Mental Health Act of 1946 (P.L. 79-487), 28-31, 34, 36, 46, 254, 256

National Mental Health Association (NMHA), 14, 27, 32

Nevada State Hospital, 62, 80, 89, 90, 102, 116, 120, 163, 227

New Madrid County, 110

Newton County, 89-90

Nodaway County, 104

North Central Missouri Mental Health Center, 108-109

Northeastern Jackson County Mental Health Center, 93, 153

Northern Ozark Mental Health Center, 116-117

Omnibus Budget Reconciliation Act of 1981 (P.L. 97-35), 52-53

Omnibus Mental Health Bill (H.B. 1724), 179-180, 198

Oregon County, 111-112

Osage County, 116

Outpatient services, 31, 34, 46, 49, 53, 58, 65-66, 71, 75-76, 82, 88, 90, 93-94, 99-103, 109, 112-116, 123-124, 129-130, 134, 138, 153, 158, 164, 171, 174, 183, 187, 189-191, 198-201, 203, 205, 209-211, 218-219, 226-227, 233, 244, 248

Ozark Center, 88-90

Ozark Community Mental Health Center, 89-90, 113

Ozark County, 112

Ozarks Medical Center Behavioral Healthcare, 112-113

Ozark Psychiatric Foundation, 89, 257

Paraprofessionals, 14, 46-47, 147, 159, 177, 206, 240-241

Park Hills Mental Health Services, 187, 191-193, 209, 212, 215

Partial hospitalization services, 46, 49, 53, 66, 103, 123, 129, 130

Partnership for Mental Health Act of 1979, 47, 171, 256

Pathways Community Behavioral Healthcare, 114-117, 193, 217-218, 221, 233, 243

Pemiscot County, 111

Perry County, 98, 134

Pettis County, 67, 115

Phelps County, 117

Pike County, 65, 88

Planned Parenthood, 154

Platte County, 91, 137

Polk County, 102

Pre-admission screening, 46, 51, 53

Prescription team, 189

President' Commission on
Mental Health, 51, 265
President's task force, 35-36,
38, 43
Prevention, 14, 22, 30, 41, 44,
45, 58, 91-94, 96, 102, 105,
108, 112, 115, 123, 128, 134,
137-139, 147, 158, 166, 171,
173, 181, 205, 213, 220-221,
231, 234, 239, 248
Privatization of state-operated
CMHCs, 60, 189-193, 210-
211, 226-227, 243-244
Psychiatric Receiving Center
(PRC), 31, 64, 66-67, 73-76
Psychosocial rehabilitation, 90,
99, 103, 109-111, 113-114,
117, 183, 188, 192, 209
Psychotropic medications, 33,
35, 75, 82, 140-141, 147, 183,
187-188, 206, 219
Public health principles, 22, 41
43, 44-45, 64, 138, 139, 234
Public Health Service Act of
1944 (P.L. 78-410), 29, 30, 64
Section 314 (d) funds, 30,
64, 69-70, 92-93, 131, 143
Public Hospital for Persons of
Insane and Disordered Minds,
13, 24
Public mental hospitals, 13, 17-
19, 24-27, 32, 38, 45-46, 51,
54-56, 59, 61, 240, 262
Pulaski County, 116
Putnam County, 108
Ralls County, 88
Randolph County, 67
Ray County, 91, 137

ReDiscover, 92-32, 149, 234
Regionalization, 174, 193-194
228, 234, 237, 243-244
Renaissance West, 94, 155
Research Mental Health
Services, 92-93, 143, 152
Reserpine, 32, 69
Responsibility for a specified
population, 14, 43, 122, 128,
137, 146, 158, 165-166, 172-
173, 205, 213, 232-234
Reynolds County, 111
Ripley County, 111
Risperdal, 187-188
Rolla Area Counseling Clinic,
117
St. Charles County, 104,
169, 170, 177-178
St. Clair County, 115
St. Francis Medical Center, 98-
99, 133-134
St. Francois County, 187
St. John's Regional Medical
Center, 89
St. Joseph State Hospital, 62,
90, 96, 102-103, 121, 141, 146
St. Louis City, 17, 18, 20,
62-67, 70-71, 79, 81-84, 87,
96-97, 169, 170, 174, 184,
187, 189, 192, 194, 199, 205,
209, 225, 240, 242, 244
St. Louis City Sanitarium, 62
St. Louis County, 62, 64, 90,
92, 106, 133, 135, 137, 186-
187, 199-203, 205, 207, 209,
232, 243, 266
St. Louis Mental Health Center,
174, 187, 189-190, 193, 205,

209-212, 226-227, 233, 244
St. Louis Regional Center, 186
St. Louis State Hospital, 63, 65, 81, 107, 169, 171, 186, 189, 199-201, 233
St. Louis University School of Medicine, 39, 63, 77
Ste. Genevieve County, 98, 134
Saline County, 67
Schuyler County, 100
Scotland County, 100
Scott County, 109
Seroquel, 187-188
Shannon County, 112
Shelby County, 100
Sheltering Arms Guidance Center, 103
Sikeston Regional Center for the Developmentally Disabled, 109-110.
Social Security Act, 54-56
  Title XVIII (Medicare), 54, 70-71, 73, 173, 220, 245
  Title XIX (Medicaid), 51, 54, 57, 71, 146, 164, 167, 173, 188-190, 202, 204, 212, 214, 220, 225-226, 239-240, 254, 258, 262
Southeast Missouri Mental Health Center, 109-111
Southeast Jackson County MHA, 149
Southeastern Jackson County Community Mental Health Center, 92
Southwest Missouri Mental Health Center, 116, 218
Standardizing rates, 184, 196
State Comprehensive Mental

Health Services Plan Act of 1986 (P.L. 99-660), 57, 224
Stoddard County, 109-110
Stone County, 101-102
Studio 410, 112
Sullivan County, 108
Swope Health Services, 95-96, 244
System redesign, 194-198
Taney County, 101-102
Texas County, 112
The privatization of state-operated CMHCs, 189-193
Thorazine, 32, 140
Transitional services, 19, 46, 51, 101, 104
Traveling clinics, 64-65, 71, 82-85, 87-89, 100, 104, 109-111, 120, 169-170, 199, 201, 232
Treating people with a mental illness in their home communities, 10, 14, 19, 46, 65, 102, 123, 128, 139, 147, 158, 176, 205, 213, 236
Tri County Counseling Center, 109-110
Tri-County Mental Health Services, 90-92, 125, 133, 136-141, 236, 243
Truman Medical Center, 92, 190, 192, 211
12,225,000 Acre Bill of 1854, 26, 30
Union-Sarah Center, 97
U.S. Congress, 12, 14, 26, 29-30, 34, 36, 38-39, 45-46, 50, 249
U.S. Public Health Service, 29-30, 64, 261

University of Missouri – Columbia, 66, 69, 74, 77, 125, 256, 266

University of Missouri – Kansas City School of Medicine, 73, 76

University of Missouri Health Care (University of Missouri Hospitals and Clinics), 191, 211, 244

Vernon County, 115

Veterans Administration, 28, 36

Warren County, 104, 169-170, 178

Washington County, 187

Washington University, 63, 65, 77-78, 80-81, 169-170, 209

Wayne County, 111

Webster County, 102

West Central Missouri Mental Health Center, 115-116

Western Jasper County MHA, 88

Western Missouri Mental Health Center, 18, 31, 36, 73, 75-76, 81, 91-93, 115, 121, 135, 143, 153-154, 190, 227, 235, 244

World War II, 22, 28-29, 31,

Worth County, 104

Wright County, 112

Yeatman District Community Corporation, 97

Yeatman Health Center, 97

Yeatman/Union-Sarah Joint Commission on Health Care, 97

Yeatman/Union-Sarah Mental Health Center, 97, 170

Zyprexa, 187-188

Appendix A

Map of Missouri Counties

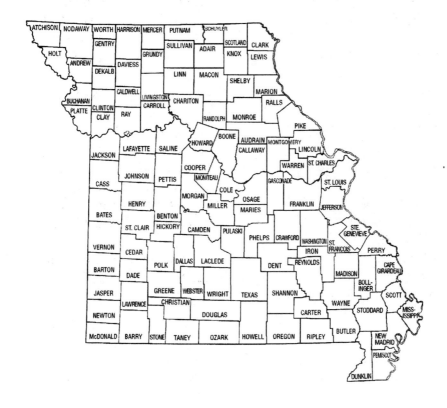

Appendix B

Recommended Readings

Barton, W.E. and Sanborn C.J. (Eds.) 1975. *An Assessment of the Community Mental Health Movement.* Lexington, MA: Lexington Books.

Beers, C.W. 1913. *A Mind that Found Itself.* New York, Longmans, Green & Co.

Bockoven, J. S. 1963. *Moral Treatment in American Psychiatry.* New York: Springer.

Caplan, G. 1964. *Principles of Preventive Psychiatry.* New York: Basic Books.

Caplan, G. 1970. *The Theory and Practice of Mental Health Consultation.* New York: Basic Books.

Cumming, E. and Cumming, J. 1957. *Closed Ranks: An Experiment in Mental Health Education.* Cambridge, MA: Harvard University Press.

Davidson, H.A. 1953. Psychiatry and the euphemistic delusion. *The American Journal of Psychiatry,* 110: 311-312.

Deutsch, A. 1948. *The Shame of the States.* New York: Harcourt, Brace and Co.

Deutsch, A. 1949. *The Mentally Ill in America.* 2nd ed. New York: Columbia University Press.

Federation of Missouri Advocates for Mental Health and Substance Abuse Services. 1999. *Reasonable Expectations for the Design and Operation of a System of Publicly Funded Psychiatric and Substance Abuse Treatment Services and Supports.* Jefferson City: Federation of Missouri Advocates for Mental Health and Substance Abuse Services.

Felix, R. H. 1967. *Mental Illness: Progress and Prospects.* New York: Columbia University Press.

Foley, H. 1975. *Community Mental Health Legislation: The*

Formative Process. Lexington, MA: D.C. Heath and Company, Lexington Books.

Goffman, E. 1961. *Asylums: Essays on the Social Situation of Mental Patients and Other Inmates.* Garden City, NY: Doubleday.

Golann, S.E. and Eisdorfer, C. (Eds.) 1972. *Handbook of Community Mental Health.* New York: Appleton-Century-Crofts.

Grob, G.N. 1991. *From Asylum to Community: Mental Health Policy in Modern America.* Princeton: Princeton University Press.

Joint Commission of Mental Illness and Health 1961. *Action for Mental Health.* New York: Basic Books.

Jones, M. 1968. *Social Psychiatry in Practice: The Idea of a Therapeutic Community.* New York: Penguin.

Kennedy, J.F. 1963. *Message of the President of the United States Relative to Mental Illness and Mental Retardation.* 88th Congress, First Session, U.S. House of Representatives Document No. 58. U.S. Government Printing Office.

Leighton, A.H. 1982. *Caring for Mentally Ill People: Psychological and Social Barriers in Historical Context.* Cambridge: Cambridge University Press.

Parad, H. 1965. *Crisis Intervention: Selected readings.* New York: Family Service Association of America.

Rochefort, D. A. 1997. *From Poorhouses to Homelessness: Policy Analysis and Mental Health Care.* 2nd ed. Westport, CT: Auburn House.

Singh, R.K.J. 1971. *Community Mental Health Consultation and Crisis Intervention.* Berkeley, CA: Book People.

Stanton, A.H. and Schwartz, M.H. 1954. *The Mental Hospital: A Study of Institutional Participation in Psychiatric Illness and Treatment.* New York: Basic Books.

Szasz, T. 1961. *The Myth of Mental Illness.* New York: Harper & Row.

Ward, M.J. 1946. *The Snake Pit.* New York: Random House.

Quick Order Form – Copy and Send

Fax orders: Fax this form toll free to: 877-862-3202
Telephone orders: 888-272-0767 (toll free)
E-mail orders: cpc@cpcontext.com
Postal orders: Causeway Publishing Company
                        P.O. Box 1248
                        Fenton, MO 63026

Please send me _____ copies of
**Made in Missouri: The Community Mental Health Movement
and Community Mental Health Centers, 1963-2003,**
*at $23.95 each, plus $3.00 per book for shipping and handling.
Add all applicable sales taxes.*

Also by Paul R. Ahr, Ph.D., M.P.A

Please send me _____ copies of **Notes for the Vigilant, the Active, the
Brave: Certain things for uncertain times**: *18 observations on the
challenges facing the Missouri Department of Mental Health and its
provider networks at the beginning of the 21st century,
at $12.50 each, plus $3.00 per book for shipping and handling.
Add all applicable sales taxes.*

By Paul R. Ahr, Ph.D., M.P.A. and Thomas B. Ahr, D.Mgt., PHR

Please send me _____ copies of
**Overturn Turnover: Why some employees leave, why some
employees stay, and ways to keep the ones who you want to stay,**
*at $14.95 each, plus $3.00 per copy for shipping and handling,
Add all applicable sales taxes.*

Name: _____

Organization: _____

Address: _____

City: _____

State/Zip: _____

Telephone: _____

e-mail: _____

Quick Order Form – Copy and Send

Fax orders:	Fax this form toll free to: 877-862-3202
Telephone orders:	888-272-0767 (toll free)
E-mail orders:	cpc@cpcontext.com
Postal orders:	Causeway Publishing Company
	P.O. Box 1248
	Fenton, MO 63026

Please send me _____ copies of
**Made in Missouri: The Community Mental Health Movement
and Community Mental Health Centers, 1963-2003,**
*at $23.95 each, plus $3.00 per book for shipping and handling.
Add all applicable sales taxes.*

Also by Paul R. Ahr, Ph.D., M.P.A

Please send me _____ copies of **Notes for the Vigilant, the Active, the
Brave: Certain things for uncertain times**: *18 observations on the
challenges facing the Missouri Department of Mental Health and its
provider networks at the beginning of the 21st century,
at $12.50 each, plus $3.00 per book for shipping and handling.
Add all applicable sales taxes.*

By Paul R. Ahr, Ph.D., M.P.A. and Thomas B. Ahr, D.Mgt., PHR

Please send me _____ copies of
**Overturn Turnover: Why some employees leave, why some
employees stay, and ways to keep the ones who you want to stay,**
*at $14.95 each, plus $3.00 per copy for shipping and handling,
Add all applicable sales taxes.*

Name: _____

Organization: _____

Address: _____

City: _____

State/Zip: _____

Telephone: _____

e-mail: _____